DEATH CAN
BE CURED

**And 99 Other
Medical Hypotheses**

DEATH CAN BE CURED

And 99 Other Medical Hypotheses

Roger Dobson

CYAN

Copyright © 2007 Cyan Communications Limited

First published in 2007 by Cyan Books, an imprint of
Cyan Communications Limited
5th floor
32–38 Saffron Hill
London ECIN 8FH
United Kingdom
Tel: +44 (0)20 7421 8145
E: sales@cyanbooks.com
www.cyanbooks.com

A CIP record for this book is available from the British Library

ISBN-13 978-1-905736-31-7
ISBN-10 1-905736-31-2

Printed in the UK by CPI Bookmarque, Croydon, CR0 4TD

Disclaimer
The theories discussed in this book are hypothetical and speculative only
and are intended solely for debate. No statement made here constitutes
medical or any other kind of advice or recommendation of any course of
action or inaction. No responsibility for any consequences, however caused,
of any acts or omissions arising from any part of this text will be accepted by
the author, *Medical Hypotheses* or Cyan Communications Limited.

For my wife Alex, our children, Jessica, Ben, Lizzie and James,
and Mum & Dad

CONTENTS

FOREWORD

MEDICAL HYPOTHESES, A JOURNAL OF medical science ideas, was
founded in 1976 by David F. Horrobin. Following David's premature death in 2003, I became editor-in-chief.

Medical Hypotheses is different in two main respects. First, it is
primarily dedicated to publishing ideas rather than experimental
and observational findings. This is very unusual in medical science,
where the vast bulk of funding and organization is devoted to
empirical research, and where analysis and theory have been
underdeveloped for many decades. Second, *Medical Hypotheses*
makes a deliberate effort to publish potentially revolutionary
ideas, even though these are less likely to turn out to be wholly
correct than the more modest improvements that make up mainstream scientific literature.

In 1976 it was extremely difficult to publish theories in medical
science, especially revolutionary ones. *Medical Hypotheses*, with its
international distribution in libraries and indexing by the major
scientific databases, was literally the only avenue through which
some researchers could reach a wider audience. Since then, with
the development of the Internet and the possibility of almost
anyone making their work available almost anywhere in the world,
the role of *Medical Hypotheses* has changed. Now, I see the journal
as providing a forum where revolutionary science meets the mainstream. Articles follow the standard scientific style and format,
but the content may be much more speculative than is allowed by
the pre-publication screening process of peer review, where ideas
must pass the test of verification according to an intrinsically con-
servative professional consensus.

Naturally enough, this means that the papers in *Medical Hypotheses* are exactly that: hypotheses, requiring further evaluation by the processes of science. However, that constraint applies to all true science. Unless it is an incremental extrapolation of standard knowledge using standard methods, science is never valid at the time of publication.

After all, peer review is not distinctive or specific to the natural sciences; it is deployed by all academic subjects, from English literature to theology. Peer review of literary criticism or systematic theology may ensure high standards, but it does not make these activities branches of the natural sciences. Instead, science is validated or refuted after publication by being tested against real-world observations. Ultimately, it is the "peer usage" criterion of how ideas stand up to testing that matters, and not peer review itself, which is little more than an expert opinion poll.

When David Horrobin handed over responsibility for the journal, he said that in his experience editorial review was the only viable way to fulfil the journal's objectives of encouraging revolutionary science, since peer review always tended to gravitate towards rejecting radical ideas as likely to prove incorrect. Like David, I have processed submissions to *Medical Hypotheses* using the same system that prevailed during the golden era of revolutionary science. In other words, the editor-in-chief takes responsibility for evaluating and choosing the content of the journal, assisted – when he thinks it will be useful – by a relatively small editorial advisory board.

Understanding the essence of science as a post-publication evaluation enables *Medical Hypotheses* to be far more adventurous than other journals. We publish ideas, not because we are confident they are correct in all respects, but because they would be important if they were correct; or because, although flawed, they might contain important insights; or because even ideas that are both incorrect and flawed can nevertheless be thought-provoking and stir debate in a way that is both useful and enlightening.

It might be imagined that a journal which operates by such

criteria would be regarded as too far beyond the pale to be worth considering; yet the mission and methods of *Medical Hypotheses* have always been endorsed by some of the most prestigious scientists. Those who have served on the editorial advisory board have included Nobel prizewinners James Black and Arvid Carlsson, Fellows of the Royal Society Sir John Eccles, Sir Roy Calne and John Ziman, and international superstars of clinical science Antonio Damasio and V. S. Ramachandran.

Furthermore, the "impact factor" of *Medical Hypotheses* – which measures the number of times on average an article is referenced in the scientific literature – currently stands at 1.3, which compares favourably with most mainstream medical journals. About 2,200 "Web of Science" articles formally reference *Medical Hypotheses* papers each year, and *Medical Hypotheses* articles are downloaded from the Internet about 26,000 times a month. These statistics make it clear that, despite its radical ambitions and unconventional methods, *Medical Hypotheses* is playing a significant role in the functioning of medical science.

I have to admit that the marvellous selection of *Medical Hypotheses* articles in *Death Can Be Cured* is oriented towards the more colourful end of the journal's spectrum. The majority of papers may indeed be somewhat bolder and more radical than usual, but this may only be apparent to the specialist. Nonetheless, every issue contains ideas of the type selected by Roger Dobson, and our authors run the full gamut from senior scientists at the world's leading universities, through people engaged at the cutting edge of clinical practice, to independent researchers in all conceivable walks of life.

My thanks are due to Roger Dobson and Cyan Books for this delightful volume, which serves as an entertaining and edifying introduction to the sometimes strange but always stimulating world of *Medical Hypotheses*.

Bruce G. Charlton
Editor-in-chief, *Medical Hypotheses*

1

NIGHT TERRORS, BIRTHMARKS AND OTHER SCIENTIFIC THEORIES

Short-sighted people are more intelligent

MYOPIA IS A MODERN EPIDEMIC. In some populations 80 per cent of young adults are short-sighted, and research suggests that in each generation over the last century there has been a significant increase in the numbers of myopics.

Children with one myopic parent are more likely to develop the condition, and the risk increases if both parents are affected, suggesting that, to some extent at least, it's genetically determined.

But if there is a gene for myopia, how has it survived evolutionary pressures? In prehistoric times, any hunter-gatherer with poor vision would not have survived long; nor would he have been an attractive proposition as a mate and family provider. So, according to evolutionary theory, the myopia genes should have perished over time. Yet, myopia is not only still with us, its prevalence is increasing at an alarming rate. How can this be?

According to researchers at Queen Mary Hospital, London and the University of Hong Kong, the myopia gene or genes survived because they have a second, more important role to play in intelligence.

It's known that academically gifted students and high achievers are more likely to be myopic, but the traditional explanation for this is that short-sightedness is simply a marker for children who read at an early age and who are therefore more likely to be brighter.

New research proposes a much more direct link between myopia and intelligence. It claims that higher intelligence and myopia go together because the growth of the brain and the eyes has a common genetic base. Crucially, though, the genetic element responsible for myopia has to be activated by an environmental trigger. The theory is that in the distant past that trigger didn't exist, so our ancestors benefited from the genetic material that brought superior intelligence, but did not have the handicap of being short-sighted.

"During human evolution, the gene was strongly selected because it facilitated the survival of our ancestors," say the researchers. "They could apply intelligence to refine their hunting, foraging, farming or herding techniques. The myopia component was of little detriment because it was not manifested in the ancestral environment and, therefore, was selectively neutral. As a result, there is a net gain in Darwinian fitness and the gene could attain a very high frequency in the human population, as reflected by the current prevalence of myopia."

But what is that environmental trigger? What today is switching on the genetic material involved in myopia?

Well, one thing that modern man does that the hunter-gathers didn't is read, and it may be reading, especially when started at a young age, that is the trigger. If that is the case, say the Hong Kong researchers, it may be possible to prevent the myopia genetic material being turned on by avoiding what they describe as unnatural eye usage during childhood:

"Early visual experiences can be controlled by discouraging intensive schooling, excessive near-work, and leisure activities associated with complex visual inputs such as television viewing and video games. Any strategies along this line must be started early and maintained to cover the whole susceptible period."

Revelations always happen on mountains

THAT BURNING BUSH AND MYSTERIOUS voice that Moses encountered on Mount Sinai may not have been a spiritual revelation after all, but a hallucination caused by spending too much time at high altitude. And when Jesus appeared to Peter, John and James in a cloud of glory on a mountainside, that too could have been a hallucination triggered by brain changes.

Researchers say that marked similarities between reports of the revelations that feature in the major religions and mountaineers' descriptions of hallucinatory experiences suggest that both may be the result of altitude effects on the brain. And it may be no coincidence that the fundamental revelations to Moses, Jesus and Mohammed, the founders of the three main monotheistic religions, occurred on mountains.

On Mount Sinai (2600 m) Moses experienced his first revelation in the form of a burning bush, and encountered the Hebrew God three more times. Jesus was transfigured on a mountain peak – possibly Mount Hermon (2841m) – and appeared in a cloud of glory. And in the Islamic tradition, Mohammed received the Qur'an while alone on Mount Hira (2000 m) through a revelation of the Archangel Gabriel.

According to the research, these revelatory experiences had many common features, including feeling and hearing a presence, seeing a figure and lights, and experiencing fear.

Similar experiences, say researchers from a number of institutions, including University Hospital, Geneva, and the Hebrew University, Jerusalem, have been reported by mountaineers.

Climbers have described the experience of feeling or hearing a presence, as well as complex visual hallucinations and body photism – an appearance of unexplained colour and bright lights. There have also been reports of out-of-body experiences, anxiety, fear and sudden temperature changes. As with the religious revelations, most of these occurred when the climbers were alone.

One theory is that two areas of the brain – the temporo-parietal junction and the prefrontal cortex – are involved. Both areas could be affected by altitude and each has been linked to changes in body perception and mystical experiences.

Another possibility is that prolonged time spent at high altitudes, especially alone, may lead to prefrontal lobe dysfunction and a loss of inhibition. Yet another suggestion is that the environmental effects of solitude in the mountains may be enough to trigger an effect on the mind.

The researchers point out that although the religious revelations occurred at moderate rather than high altitudes, that can be sufficient to trigger revelation-like experiences. Mountain sickness, for example, has been reported in some people at even low to moderate altitudes.

"These different findings might suggest that the frequent appearance of the mountain metaphor in revelation experiences of mystics might be related to interference with functional and neural mechanisms," say the researchers. "Based on these findings we suggest that exposure to altitudes might contribute to the induction of revelation experiences and might further our understanding of the mountain metaphor in religion."

Fat people *really* are more jolly

FOR CENTURIES FATNESS has been associated with jollity. From Father Christmas to Falstaff, Billy Bunter to Benny Hill, anyone who has visibly eaten more than their fair share is invariably portrayed as being funny, jolly and pretty much content with life.

Everyone knows that in literature, opera and the movies heroes and heroines are slim and fat people are funny. Lean men get the girls; fat men get the laughs. But is it the same in real life? Are fat people happier, or is it just media stereotyping?

According to research by psychologists at Lakehead University, Canada the jolly fat hypothesis may be true, at least for women. Not only have they found a link, they suggest a mechanism too – oestrogen. They have put forward the idea that body fat protects women against negative mood. In other words, the fatter a woman is, the less depressed she gets.

In the two-part research, the team looked at body mass index (a measure that takes into account weight and height) and compared it with mood in a group of young women.

What they found was that the higher the BMI and body size, the fewer symptoms of depression, anxiety and negative mood. In fact, the most depressed women were all thin, while the largest were the least miserable.

The researchers say that, statistically, the connection between weight and mood they found was as big as the known link between stress and health.

For an explanation, they turned to biochemical research and that suggested the possibility of a link between oestrogen and mood, and the brain chemical serotonin, the target of widely prescribed antidepressant drugs. Very potent oestrogens are primarily found in fatty tissue, which suggests that heavier women may have higher levels of oestrogen than thin women.

If there is such a hormonal link, there should also be differences across the monthly cycle in both mood and weight. They found there were two occasions when body size and negative affect were most highly linked – day 11 and days 24 and 25 of the monthly cycle. Both occur around periods of higher oestrogen levels.

"Our findings suggest an association between body size and mood," say the researchers. "Women with larger BMIs experience fewer symptoms of depression, anxiety, and negative affect than women with smaller BMIs. Consistent with the 'jolly fat' hypothesis, women with greater body fat may experience fewer and less severe negative affect and mood symptoms than their slimmer peers. Preliminary results suggest that oestrogen may have an effect on both body fat storage and negative affect. The cyclical release of oestrogen may also have effects on negative affect in women."

Nightmares can kill you

THE YOUNGISH MAN, WELL-BUILT and seemingly healthy, didn't know it, but he'd just eaten his last supper. Two hours later he went to bed and fell asleep, but within minutes he was moving vigorously around the bed. He was agitated, groaning, shouting and coughing, but all attempts to wake him failed and a short time later he was dead.

A traditional belief among Filipinos is that people in this state die from nightmares. There have been reports from Vietnam, Kampuchea, Laos, Japan and the USA of many similar sudden deaths. They are known as Sudden Unexplained Nocturnal Death in the United States, *Bangungut* in the Philippines and *Pokkuri* in Japan. In these cases post mortems usually only reveal signs of acute heart failure, but the underlying cause of such dramatic, traumatic deaths is unknown. The victims have rarely had a diagnosis of heart disease during their life and are almost always in good health. So what killed them?

Researchers at the Departments of Ophthalmology and Neurosciences of the University of California at San Diego suggest the victims were experiencing night terrors, a sort of super-nightmare. Night terrors are different from run-of-the-mill, spooky nightmares. They occur in deep sleep and even if the dreamer is awakened, the terrors may still be experienced for another 15 minutes or so. Usually the sufferer has no recall of the dream content, and some research suggests there may well be none – no scary monsters, no ghosts. What these people are experiencing is primitive, raw fear.

Children who have night terrors, which occur mostly between the ages of 5 and 7, are usually described as screaming, sitting bolt upright, eyes wide open and with a look of fear and panic. Similar features appear in adults, at least in those who do wake, and it's been estimated that around 4 per cent of nightmares are actually night terrors.

The research shows that among those who died, deaths occurred on average 3.5 hours after the start of sleep. In most cases the first signs were groans, gasps or very laboured breathing. The heart rate can increase to 170 beats a minute within 15–45 seconds of the start of a night terror attack, which probably represents one of the greatest accelerations of the heart possible, even greater than those associated with violent exercise or orgasm.

Some post mortems have shown undiagnosed abnormalities in the heart of the deceased. One of the most common findings is heart arrhythmia, which would affect the pumping of the heart. These findings point to those who died having undetected heart problems which were triggered by the dramatic effects on the heart of the raw fear experienced in night terrors.

"We propose that night terror occurring in a patient with an underlying cardiac defect can on occasion culminate in sudden death and may explain the development of a fatal arrhythmia in Sudden Unexplained Nocturnal Death," they say.

Birthmarks are proof of reincarnation

WHEN RESEARCHERS BEGAN INVESTIGATING CHILDREN who claimed to remember a previous life, the findings themselves bordered on the supernatural. Among those children who also had phobias, the cause of the fear was nearly always found to be the same as the mode of death they claimed to have witnessed in a prior existence. A child who claimed to remember a life that ended in drowning, for example, was more likely to have a phobia of being immersed in water. In fact, the researchers found that 6 out of 10 children who remembered a death by drowning had a phobia of water. A similar trend was found for snakes and guns.

There are many reports of children talking about a previous life, but relatively few have been investigated in any detail. Where there has been any kind of inquiry, the main method, says the report from a researcher at the University of Virginia, has been interviews with parents or carers of the child and with people connected with the deceased person concerned, backed up by post-mortem reports.

According to the Virginia research, in the majority of cases investigated – 67 per cent of 856 cases in one series – the dead person who had been named by the child could be identified, and the facts of their life and death matched the child's statements.

The report says that many disorders or abnormalities seen in medicine and psychology cannot be fully explained by genetics and environmental influences. As examples it cites phobias in early infancy, gender identity disorder, differences in temperament seen soon after birth and unusual birthmarks.

The report suggests that what it calls the hypothesis of previous lives can explain a number of these phenomena which defy more rational explanation.

Take phobias. In 387 children who claimed to remember a previous life, phobias occurred in 141 (36 per cent) of them. In many cases, say the researchers, the child developed the phobia before he or she had spoken about a previous life. In one study, 56 per cent of parents were not able to explain how their child had developed a phobia of water.

The report says that many children who claim to remember a previous life also have birthmarks that correspond to the position of wounds in the life apparently remembered. Out of 895 cases investigated, from nine different countries and cultures, 309 (35 per cent) had such birthmarks. The site of the birthmarks and wounds or other marks on the body of the deceased was verified by post-mortem reports.

"I suggest that the phobias of water in these children, even though they had never mentioned a previous life, might have derived from death by drowning in one," says the report. "I believe that previous lives may contribute to the understanding of the location of some birthmarks." It adds, "The investigation of these cases has progressed to the point where the hypothesis of previous lives offers at least a plausible interpretation of many cases, and for some it seems to be the strongest one."

Global warming reduces fertility

ICEBERGS MELTING, SEA LEVELS RISING, islands disappearing, tropical temperatures in Yorkshire, vineyards in Scotland … there's no end to the changes being predicted due to the effects of global warming. But could one of its most significant effects already be happening and have gone unnoticed? Is global warming to blame for the worldwide drop in fertility and birth rates?

According to research by a team at Columbia University College of Physicians and Surgeons, New York and Columbia-Presbyterian Medical Center, the evidence points that way: "The results of our analyses are consistent with the underlying premise that temperature change affects fertility and suggests that human fertility may have been influenced by change in environmental temperatures," they say.

There is no doubt that fertility has declined in the industrial-ized world and, to a lesser extent, in developing countries. While social and economic changes may account for some of the change, it does not explain it all. Nor does it explain why other research is consistently finding that the sperm count is going down in a number of countries.

The New York team say the decline is real, and that by 2040 some nations will have negative population growth – in other words, their populations will fall.

In their research, the team used birth data from 19 countries for the last century and compared these with figures from the National Aeronautics and Space Administration (NASA) on global air temperature changes over the same period. The results show that in each of the 19 countries there was a marked decline in the birth rate over the century. In the USA, the birth rate dropped from 30 births per 1,000 people to 10 over the course of the century. A similar drop was found in most industrialized countries. Over the same period temperatures went up. "We found a remarkably strong inverse relationship between changes in temperature and birth rates in all 19 countries," they say. Even when they took into account social, cultural and economic changes, the link with temperature persisted.

The researchers say that a number of studies have suggested a link between fertility and temporary temperature changes. For example, in hot countries, fertility varies with the seasons, with sperm counts lowest in the summer and highest in the winter. Laboratory research has confirmed that increases in scrotal temperature can reduce fertility.

"Our analysis leads us to believe that long-term changes in air temperature could influence human fertility," say the researchers. "Similar to transient environmental temperature change, long-term environmental temperature change may mediate fertility by changes in sperm counts. It is certainly possible that as a result of global air temperature changes, sperm counts may have fluctuated, thereby affecting birth rates."

They add, "If the relationship we found between temperature change and fertility is correct, then a drop in global temperatures may actually result in an increase in human fertility."

.

Showers are bad for the brain

ON THE FACE OF IT, having a shower seems a pretty healthy thing to do. It gets rid of dirt, bacteria and toxins, opens the skin pores, cleans the hair and has a general feel-good effect on mood.

But what if there was something nasty in the water? What if it formed itself into tiny aerosol droplets, and that as you soaped and sang, these mini-particles were travelling up your nose and into the brain? And what if you and millions of others were at risk?

The suspect is manganese, a metallic element that gets into water after contact with rocks and minerals in the ground. It's a natural compound and it's also found in low levels in foods, such as green vegetables, tea and cereals.

Its presence in water has been investigated a number of times, but in most research the levels found in drinking water have been judged to be too small to have an effect on health. But it's also known that when high levels are inhaled rather than drunk, it can have a disastrous effect. Occupational health research shows that when miners and battery workers inhale manganese, they can develop manganism, a condition similar to Parkinson's disease. Symptoms, it's reported, include lethargy, tremor, mental disturbances and even death.

Researchers at Wake Forest University School of Medicine, North Carolina say that while agencies have calculated safe levels for eating, drinking and inhaling manganese, no one has looked at the effects on the central nervous system from inhaling aerosols while showering in manganese-contaminated water.

"At first glance this may seem to be a trivial delivery vector," they say. "Nonetheless, extrapolating animal data suggests that it may actually be a serious public health consideration." Compared to eating and drinking, inhaling is far more effective at delivering manganese to the brain. The first cranial nerve in the nose offers relatively open access to the central nervous system, one that bypasses the protective blood–brain barrier. Research on animals, the researchers say, shows manganese can get around the blood–brain barrier and pass directly into the central nervous system.

The report adds that any manganese that does get through to the brain may have a cumulative effect, and it's suggested that some groups, including the elderly, pregnant women and people with iron-deficiency anaemia, are at increased risk from absorbed manganese.

Calculations show that a decade of showering in contaminated water can result in higher doses than those that have been reported to cause a build-up of deposits of manganese in the brains of rats.

"If future studies uphold the extrapolations that we have made, these results have profound implications for the health of the nation and the world," they say. "If our results are confirmed, regulatory agencies must rethink existing manganese drinking water standards. In the USA, potentially 8.7 million people are exposed to manganese levels that our model suggests might cause brain accumulation."

Small people can save the world

FOR CENTURIES, HEIGHT HAS BEEN one of the most sought-after human traits. It's been associated with intelligence, fertility, better job prospects, longevity and good health. What's more, we have been getting much taller, especially over the last 200 years. In the twentieth century, the average height of each new generation in much of Western Europe and the USA has increased by almost an inch. The Japanese have increased their height by up to five inches since the end of the Second World War when they adopted a Western lifestyle and diet.

But has it gone too far? Is height becoming an individual and world problem? Are tall people consuming disproportionate amounts of resources that could eventually bring about the extinction of man?

According to a report based on more than two decades' research, things are potentially so bad that the time may have come to change children's diets to reduce their growth potential.

"In spite of admiring greater height, a world population of increasing height and body-weight is a major threat to our environment, health and survival," say researchers from Reventropy Associates, San Diego and the University of California. "We need to minimize our demands on the earth by controlling the number of people and their average size." The authors are convinced that failure to do so will inevitably result in deterioration in the quality of life and humanity's chances for long-term survival. They add, "We believe that smaller body size can be attained through scientifically controlled caloric restriction that maximizes the health of children while reducing their growth potential. However, severe caloric restriction should not be employed during pregnancy or before the age of two years. Children would have to be monitored by physicians to provide increases in calorie or nutrient levels when indicated."

An energy-restricted diet that provides all the necessary nutrients has been shown to produce smaller animals that are much healthier, lose less mental functioning with age and have longer than normal life-spans.

If changes are not made, the implications seem dire. According to the report, increased height and weight have a huge impact on resources. A 20 per cent increase in height in the USA, for example, would mean about 130 million tons of additional food would be needed to feed the taller population. Taller people would require about 180 million more acres of farmland to supply their needs, and fresh water needs would go up by about 86 trillion gallons a year. Bigger buildings and cars would require the use of 1.2 billion tons a year of natural resources, including aluminium, copper and cement. Energy needs would increase by 40 quadrillion British thermal units a year. And a 20 per cent taller US population would produce an additional three billion tons of carbon dioxide, the major source of global warming, and generate 80 million tons more garbage.

"If we scale our civilization to accommodate our larger bodies, almost everything would cost more. Since we would need more energy, water, and various materials, structures, transportation, energy, food, water, drugs and medical care would cost more to produce, transport or store. A typical coast-to-coast airplane flight would cost an additional $33,000 because fewer people would be able to fit into current size airplanes."

The researchers say the benefits of smaller humans include less pollution of the atmosphere, land and water, as well as improved health and longevity through improved nutrition. There would also be better mental health and social order with the elimination of height prejudice for both short and tall people. Most importantly, there would be a reduced risk of a mass extinction in the near future.

"Based on the material presented, it is hoped that scientific and political leaders will recognize the risks of increasing body size on the future quality of life and survival of humanity," they say.

The date you will die can be calculated

THE ONLY CERTAINTY IN LIFE is death. But exactly when that moment comes varies widely among individuals, countries and races. In Botswana, for example, the average lifespan is around 35, while in affluent Andorra it's in the mid-eighties. Lifespan also varies widely among families living in the same country and from the same race and culture. While the average lifespan in the UK is in the seventies and eighties, some families have members who live well into the nineties, while other families struggle to survive to retirement age.

Is it all down to luck or is it genetic inheritance that determines our sell-by-date? And if the date of our death is fixed, is it possible to find out when it will be?

Yes, according to research at Gifu University, Japan, the date can, in theory, be calculated, and the formula itself is quite simple. It's called total immediate ancestral longevity (TIAL) and all you have to do is add up the ages at death of your six last relatives – mother, father and maternal and paternal grandparents – and divide the total by six.

That gives you your likely lifespan at birth. The only snag is that while the likely date of death may be pencilled into your DNA, it is also influenced by what you do during your life. Smoke 50 cigarettes a day and any genetic edge for longevity is likely to go up in smoke. What's more, you may reduce the life expectancy of future generations of your family. But eat a good diet, exercise regularly and avoid unsavoury activities, people and substances and you may live longer than your blueprint suggests.

To test the accuracy of TIAL, the researchers calculated scores for eminent scientists, including Charles Darwin, Albert Einstein and Irene Joliot Curie.

The TIAL scores for Einstein, Darwin, Curie were 390, 378, and 372 respectively, all considerably lower than the 477 of Jeanne Calment, the French woman who died in 1997 at the oldest authenticated age of 122 years and 164 days

The report says that since Darwin and Einstein exceeded their adjusted TIAL, nearly 14 per cent of their lifespan may have been the result of a good environment. In the case of Irene Curie, her father, Pierre, died in an accident at the age of 46, and her mother, Marie, also had a premature death at the age of 66 due to excessive workplace radioactive exposure. Irene Curie's TIAL score is 62 years. But she died four years short of that, at the age of 58 years, also due, at least in part, to excessive radioactive exposure.

The message from the report is that TIAL will tell you how long you will live if you have an average lifestyle. Live well and you will eke out a few more years, but pick up bad habits and you'll lose years.

"TIAL score is a convenient and easily quantifiable longevity parameter which anyone interested in determining his or her longevity can use to estimate a tentative number," says the report.

Jet lag triggers mental illness

THOUSANDS SUFFER THE SYMPTOMS of jet lag every day. Insomnia, fatigue, lack of concentration, indigestion, memory problems, irritability and exhaustion are all experienced by those who travel at speed across three or more time zones, especially when the flight is eastbound.

Jet lag is caused by disruption of the body's circadian rhythm or "body clock" which is involved in the timing of routines like eating and sleeping. For most people, the symptoms disappear in hours or at most a few days ... or do they?

According to researchers at the Hebrew University and Hadassah Medical School, Israel, there may be a more sinister side to jet lag. They say the possibility of a connection between jet lag and psychiatric disorder seems to have been underestimated and suggest it could trigger existing or new cases of affective disorders, a group of conditions that include depression, anxiety disorder, panic attacks and various phobias. It might also be involved in schizophrenia.

"There is strong evidence relating affective disorders with circadian rhythm abnormalities," they say. "It can be hypothesized that in predisposed individuals jet lag may play a role in triggering exacerbation or even *de novo* affective disorders. Furthermore, we propose the possibility that psychosis and even schizophrenia can be elicited by jet lag."

There are, they say, a number of examples of psychotic symptoms occurring during long-distance trips, including cases of transit paranoid reaction, a condition blamed on changes of environment, unfamiliar surroundings, the presence of strangers and a sense of isolation.

Results from an analysis of 359 people referred for psychiatric examination from Kennedy International Airport show that around 38 per cent had symptoms of paranoid schizophrenia, while others had manic depressive psychosis, psychotic depressive reaction and neuroses. Other research has, say the researchers, shown differences in levels of depression between east- and west-bound travellers.

Just how jet lag triggers new episodes of mental illness or even the illness itself is not clear, but the hormone melatonin could be the villain.

Secreted by the pineal gland deep inside the brain, melatonin is a key player in the regulation of the circadian rhythm and helps the body know when it is time to sleep and when to wake up. In synthetic form, as a supplement, it's widely used in some countries to combat the symptoms of jet lag itself.

But changes to the circadian rhythm and melatonin secretion abnormalities have also been linked to a number of mental disorders, say the researchers, and they cite studies suggesting that abnormal melatonin metabolism may be directly related to schizophrenia. It's also suggested that sleep deprivation affects melatonin production and may be linked to mania.

"In view of the ever-increasing numbers of long-distance travellers each year, among them many mental patients, there is a clear and urgent need for well-documented and controlled studies of this issue," say the researchers. "Clinical indications suggest that jet lag is a possible trigger in the exacerbation of existing affective disorders and in the appearance of mood disturbances in predisposed persons."

2

CHINS, BEER BELLIES AND EAR WAX

Why humans are not furry

JUST WHY MAN ALONE AMONG the primates lacks a protective coat of fur has puzzled scientists for years. Most theories suggest the loss of body hair some time during evolution is down to survival of the fittest, and that hairlessness increased fitness and gave man an advantage in hot, sunny Africa. But as New Jersey-based Judith Rich Harris points out, other mammals of similar size, including baboons, chimpanzees, gorillas, gazelles and leopards, have managed to survive pretty well in Africa without shedding body hair.

She suggests the loss of human body hair is not due to a Darwinian selection process, but the consequence of parental selection. Babies born with body hair were killed by their parents so that the gene or genes involved in body hair all but died out.

It's argued that infanticide as a method of birth control in premodern societies gave parents the power to exert an influence on the course of human evolution by deciding whether to keep or abandon a newborn. Harris puts forward the idea that modern man, and maybe his immediate predecessor, were the only naked primates in man's evolutionary line, and that *Homo erectus* and Neanderthals were as hairy as any other ape. It's suggested that Neanderthals could never have survived in Ice Age Europe and Asia without a thick coat of fur.

Some force other than selection on the basis of fitness has been at work and that force, Harris suggests, is culture. Modern man, wanting to distance himself from furry animals, adopted the belief that they, the hairless ones, were people and that anything with fur was an animal and prey.

Once the Orwell-like idea "hairlessness good, hairiness bad" became part of their culture, parental selection may, it's argued, have eliminated hairiness very quickly. As Harris puts it, "Any infant born too hairy would have elicited an 'ugh' response. In all likelihood, it would have been killed or abandoned at birth. A gene for hairiness would have been, in effect, lethal."

And such genes do exist, Harris says, and she cites the example of the rare congenital condition hypertrichosis universalis, which causes extensive body hair. She suggests we may all still have the gene for hairiness but that it's no longer active. Her theory not only provides an explanation for relatively hairless man, it may also offer a reason for the sudden demise of Neanderthals. If they were furry, as she suggests they were, they would have been considered prey to superior modern man.

"If I am correct in hypothesizing that Neanderthals were as furry as the other mammals, then this hypothesis would provide an explanation for their disappearance, shortly after *Homo sapiens* appeared on the scene. To a hungry human, a hairy Neanderthal would be seen as prey," she says.

"The Neanderthals, I propose, disappeared from Europe and Asia for the same reason that the mammoths disappeared – we ate them. We won the battle for the possession of Europe and Asia – a battle between two different species of meat-eaters – because we had better brains and a better tool-kit. We are here and the Neanderthals are not because we were better predators than they were."

The purpose of ear wax

ACCORDING TO THE "AQUATIC APE HYPOTHESIS", human ancestors once lived in a watery habitat. That's why, say supporters of the theory, most other land mammals have no conscious control over their breathing, while humans do. The voluntary control we have is, they say, comparable to that of semi-aquatic mammals which need to inhale air before they dive.

Over the years the theory has been attacked as unscientific and too vague, and even ridiculed. But according to research in Belgium, modern humans have many rudimentary characteristics that support the theory. Noses, for example, are perfectly designed to stop water getting into the lungs while swimming, and hair is ideally aligned for swimming. And why do we have many more fat cells than land animals of a similar size? Could it be residual blubber from our seagoing days?

What's more, says the research report, many common diseases and conditions may have their origins in our aquatic or semi-aquatic past, including sleep apnoea, acne, alopecia, dandruff, rhinophyma, myopia and osteoarthritis.

Take arthritis and varicose veins, for example. Most of us will suffer at some time from degenerative joint disease or osteoarthritis, and one in three adults will get varicose veins. Could it be that these disorders were less common in a watery habitat and that we suffer because there is no longer a counter-pressure of surrounding water?

And look at asthma. It's unknown in apes, but according to the research, seals have broncho-constriction while diving, and deep-diving mammals close the bronchi completely during diving.

Then there is short-sightedness. In myopia the eyeball is too long, and at first sight there doesn't seem to be any obvious advantage to it. But according to the research, closer scrutiny suggests a maritime link. Whales, seals and penguins are all nearsighted outside the water because they need the best vision for use in water. Thus myopia, it's argued, is an adaptation to the different refractive power of water.

Obesity too has links to a previous watery life. According to the research, all sea mammals are thick-bellied, and in an aquatic habitat, the complications of obesity would have been far less because the fat would be supported by water.

And then there's ear wax. When it's wet it absorbs water and swells, and can block the ear canal. So when semi-aquatic man went into the water, any ear wax would swell and keep out infections, but man would not have lost hearing because the wax would have conducted sound waves.

"The abundance of ex-aquatic features and ex-aquatic diseases in man is an indication for a rather recent semi-aquatic phase in our evolutionary history," says the report. "The ancestors of *Homo erectus* – perhaps no longer than two million years ago – were highly aquatic."

Hearing voices could save your life

THE LONDON HOUSEWIFE, WITH NO history of mental or physical illness, was in her thirties when she suddenly began to hear a voice. It was neither a demon nor an angel, and the message relayed to her was not religious, spiritual or philosophical. In fact, there was only ever one theme to the message: "Have a brain scan."

Referred to a psychiatrist for tests, she was prescribed antidepressants and although the voice was silenced for a very short time, it soon returned as clear and as specific as before. After several months, and mainly to reassure her, a scan was carried out.

To the surprise of her doctors, the scan showed that she had a meningioma, a tumour of the meninges, the protective membranes around the brain and spinal cord. It was more than an inch in diameter and was subsequently excised by surgeons.

When the woman awoke from the anaesthesia after the surgery, the voice apparently came one last time. This time the message was different. It simply said "Goodbye" and was never heard again.

Paranormal phenomena like this, events that cannot be explained by science, are regularly reported in medical literature, and surveys suggest that most people have at least one paranormal belief they hold to be true, with telepathy and extra-sensory perception the most popular.

Could there be any substance to some of the paranormal claims? Do we scoff simply because science has yet to come up with an explanation? After all, those who first thought the earth was round and those who suggested that it wasn't the centre of the universe were laughed at or persecuted.

In his research, Robert Bobrow, of the Department of Family Medicine, at Health Sciences Center, Stony Brook, New York, reviewed paranormal cases that have been reported, mainly by doctors, in medical literature. Those he reviewed included apparently successful cases of witchcraft, distant healing, auditory hallucinations, self-predicted death, lycanthropy (the delusion of being a wolf), speaking an unlearned foreign language under hypnosis and multiple cases of children who talk about an unknown, deceased person. In each case doctors were unable to come up with a logical explanation for what had happened. In a witchcraft case, for example, a 28-year-old Philippine-American woman who was diagnosed with lupus was unwilling to take increasing amounts of medication and returned to the village where she was born. There, the witchdoctor removed a curse placed on her by a previous suitor and she returned home three weeks later apparently cured.

Bobrow says it is important to keep an open mind: "The inability of existing paradigms to explain these observations does not negate them; rather, it elucidates a need for more research. We accept that the earth is round. Yet the earth appears flat, and was believed for eons to be so. We accept radio and television and cellular phones, whereby a sight or sound is transformed into an electromagnetic waveform which travels at the speed of light instantaneously and is then reassembled and reproduced exactly. Yet we do not accept the idea that a thought or perception is capable of emanating from one brain to another, as we lack the supporting physics. Considering that even 150 years ago, our modern technologies would have been inconceivable, it is naïve to think we are finished learning about the universe."

The reason for chins

THEY COME IN ALL SORTS of shapes and sizes, and some are bigger than others. Some stick out while others recede, a few have dimples and many have spots, but by and large, the chin is a universal feature that is unique to modern man.

But what's it for? Ancient man and Neanderthals didn't have one, and the first chin did not appear until the arrival of *Homo sapiens*. So what's the evolutionary purpose of a chin? Ears, nose, eyes, lips, even eyebrows and eyelashes all have obvious functions, but chins?

Until now, there have been two main theories. The first is that it has no function at all, it just happened, a sort of evolutionary structural blip, while the second suggests it helps with the chewing of food. The problem with the second theory is that the chin emerged at a time when the use of teeth for ripping raw food was not increasing, and may in fact have been declining.

To investigate other theories, dentists at Otago University, Dunedin, New Zealand constructed three-dimensional models of a human mandible with and without a chin and measured all the forces and angles that are experienced by the jaw in everyday use. They looked at the loading on muscles and bones from various activities to see what could have led to the evolution of the chin. Their research showed that when a tongue contracts at a 45-degree angle in a mandible without a chin, there are increased stresses and strains concentrated at exactly the point where the chin would be.

It's known that bone can change shape in response to stress, so it is possible that the chin evolved over time in response to changing stresses and pressures from the tongue. But what was so different about the tongue of modern man compared to all those who had gone before? They all had tongues, so what was special about *Homo sapiens*? The answer is simple – speech.

The researchers say it's thought that language first made its appearance among our common ancestors 50,000 years ago, which coincides with the emergence of the human chin. With the development of speech came a new repertoire of movements of the tongue and lips, generating different strains and stresses in the mouth and jaw which, say the researchers, resulted in the adaptive changes of bone to form the chin.

The tongue is designed for fast contraction and its rapid acceleration during speech generates highly repetitive forces at the area now occupied by the chin.

"We conclude that the forces generated during speech rather than those generated during mastication, shaped the chin of anatomically modern humans," say the researchers. "We propose that strong, repetitive contractions of the tongue ... demanded by the newly acquired facility of spoken language in modern humans, resulted in an adaptive remodelling of the chin." They add, "This provides a new perspective on the generation of the chin and importantly suggests that its appearance may be related to the development of the human language."

Humour increases survival

AMONG HUMANS A SENSE of humour is almost universal. Some may be more developed than others, some may be fast and others slow, but we pretty much all have one. But why? There is no evidence that any other species has a sense of humour, so how come we ended up with one, and why is it pleasurable?

Because it is found in every culture and ethnic group, humour must have appeared early in the evolution of human beings. If so, there must be a survival advantage to having a good sense of humour.

Many other enjoyable things in life, like eating and sex, are easily explained from an evolutionary point of view. Individuals who don't enjoy eating and dislike sex are clearly less likely to procreate and pass on their genes. Yet there is no such obvious explanation for humour − or is there?

What we find funny, the report says, is not so much what is physically happening as our ability to look into the mind of the butt of the humour as he realizes what is happening. And in the ancient world those who had the best sense of humour were better able to survive and become leaders of the pack.

"Humour comes when we see and understand the subject as he reacts to the changed situation. That is, the actual source of amusement is our observation of the resolution in the mind of the subject of the collision between old perception and new reality," the report says. "The Mind Reading Hypothesis argues that what's funny is our observation and understanding of the wheels turning inside his head. Humour comes from our appreciation of the conscious mind being forced to deal with the new set of circumstances."

That mind-reading ability, the reports suggests, makes it a useful thing for early man to have had because those with the keenest sense of humour would have had the edge on others.

Research shows that people who initiate humour are seen as more sociable. Low-ranking group members can boost their standing, says the report, by being the first to recognize and make fun of the idiosyncrasies of the leader. Everyone has seen, for example, what the class clown can do to a teacher.

"Those of our ancestors who could read the thoughts of others and get pleasure from being able to interpret their expressions would have achieved power within the community," says the report. "That power would have translated into a strong selective advantage. The conclusion is that a sense of humour evolved and spread throughout the human population because of the competitive advantage that it gave over those who didn't have it."

Babies suck to avoid asthma

FOR THE FIRST TWO to three years of life, babies suck almost anything.

In the first 12 months, the most intense period for sucking or avid mouthing, just about everything within grabbing distance will find its way into the mouth. Exactly why that should be is not clear. In evolutionary terms it's a trait that should have disappeared because it appears to carry no survival advantage, and has, in fact, a distinct disadvantage. In the USA, between one and 18 out of every 100,000 infants die each year due to accidental poisoning, and four out of 100,000 lose their lives choking on foreign objects.

In order for such a trait to survive, there should be some positive side to avid mouthing that outweighs the downside of such high-risk behaviour. Natural selection has it that high-cost behaviour survives either because it is an unavoidable by-product of another, desired feature, or it has a benefit which may not be immediately obvious that is greater than the potential cost.

Not surprisingly, Sigmund Freud's view on avid mouthing was that it was all down to sensual gratification arising from the mouth being the sole source of nourishment. A subsequent and widely accepted theory is that babies put objects in their mouths as a way of exploring and learning about their environment. But critics say that the benefits of such information-gathering are not in proportion to the potentially high cost of the risks involved. They also say that babies and toddlers use other ways to collect such information which are much less costly.

The theory put forward by anthropologists at the University of California is that sucking has a much more important and vital role, and that it may be a way of protecting babies from diseases as diverse as asthma and rheumatoid arthritis.

At birth, the immune system is working but still developing. The hypothesis is that by putting items in their mouths, babies are educating their immature immune systems to identify good and bad bugs. All this is done, it's argued, under the protective umbrella of breast-feeding which protects the baby from anything really nasty.

By exposing themselves to random and diverse toxins, germs and bacteria on the items they put into their mouths, the babies are in effect calibrating or priming their immune system. The cost of failing to calibrate properly could be an increased risk of allergy, asthma and other autoimmune disorders.

The whole process has to be completed under the protection of breast-feeding. It is known that breast-feeding does offer protection and it has been shown to reduce the incidence of diarrhoea, pneumonia and ear infections in babies. Some research also shows that orphans without a wet nurse have higher mortality rates.

"We propose that mouthing serves to proactively expose the naive gastrointestinal tract to environmental antigens and bacteria while under the sheltering umbrella of breast-feeding," say the researchers. "The immune system has a critical period of calibration, in which the neonate adjusts its investment in the immune system to reflect the environment into which it has been born. Failure to accurately expose the immune system to sufficient antigens within the critical time period may entail significant costs, including increased risk of allergy, asthma, and autoimmune disorders." They add, "Although allergy, asthma, and autoimmune diseases are mostly disorders of Western and urban settings, changing ideals of cleanliness in developing countries may yet greatly increase their prevalence."

Beer bellies protect men in old age

HOWEVER GOOD YOU ARE at dieting, however keen you are to exercise and keep fit, as soon as you hit your thirties, the pounds start piling on.

In the early teenage years, at least until the recent obesity epidemic, weight stayed pretty much the same whatever we ate, and however little exercise we did. But beyond the twenties, the average Western adult starts to get wider and thicker, putting on 3–5 kg a decade, so that by the age of 50, the scales are showing, on average, an extra 10–15 kg. Then, after 60, it's rare for any more weight to be added.

Obesity epidemic aside, that overall pattern has been pretty much the same in every Western country, and while there have been a number of theories, there is no consensus on what could explain it.

While some say it could just be down to men becoming less active, or eating and drinking more as they get older, researchers at the Schneider Children's Medical Centre, Israel suggest that it's all down to what they call the "Young Hunter Hypothesis". Their suggestion is that age-related weight gain is a major driving force behind human longevity. They argue that the muscle of the young hunter is turned into fat stores for the non-working, non-hunting older man to survive on in old age.

In ancient times, the food providers, the hunters, needed to be very muscular for long, hard and dangerous hunting expeditions. To develop the necessary muscles, body fat was diverted from the lower limbs, and energy was targeted at bulking up the muscles.

But when men reached the end of their hunting careers, there was a redirection of metabolic processes towards energy conservation in anticipation of ageing. In fact, there is an average drop of about 15 per cent in muscle mass after the age of 30, and a gradual increase in levels of fat, particularly around the central area.

According to the Israeli hypothesis, the muscle loss means fuel that previously went to the muscle now ends up as fat in the older man. No longer able to hunt for food, those reserves were designed to last him through old age, and their evolutionary purpose, it's suggested, may be to allow him to live long enough to see his family grow up. That may explain why men do not usually put on any more weight after their sixties, the age at which the children would have become independent.

"The continuous individual weight gain during adult life in modern affluent societies seems to have its evolutionary roots in human biologic and cultural traits," say the researchers. "Weight gain is an adaptive process engineered to compensate for adult muscle mass loss guaranteeing survival and longevity." They add, "Our hypothesis is based on the assumption that age-related weight gain evolved as a protective means to ensure sufficient energy stores for basic metabolic needs during late adulthood, when energy-consuming activities are curtailed due to age-dependent muscle mass loss."

Why winter swimmers don't shiver

WE'VE ALL SEEN THEM. Every Christmas and New Year's Day, while we are eating and drinking too much, they're out there for the first swim of the year, up to their necks in freezing water.

Many of them seem not to be in the first flush of youth and a high proportion are in the age band where the risk of heart disease and stroke is beginning to peak. So how do they do it? What's the secret of winter swimming?

For most of us swimming is about holidays, hotels, sunny resorts, warm water and fun, but for some, regular swimming in cold water is best, and members of the growing number of Polar

Bear clubs in the northern hemisphere believe it gives them energy and keeps them healthy.

There is no doubt that conventional swimming is healthy. It builds up cardiovascular fitness as well as muscle strength. It's also been estimated that we burn up three calories for every pound of weight for each mile we swim. So, if you weigh around 150 pounds, you could use around 900 calories in an hour of intense, fast swimming.

But while swimming in moderately warm water is healthy, cold water can be very unhealthy for some. According to researchers at the University of Ioannina, Greece, there are 400–1,000 deaths associated with swimming in cold water in Britain each year. The main causes of death are heart problems and stroke.

Immersion in cold water results in immediate and long-term physical changes. There is an increase in metabolism, and shivering thermogenesis kicks in – thermal energy is produced by muscle contractions as we shiver. If shivering fails to work, as little as 30 minutes exposure to low temperatures can lead to hypothermia.

According to the research, the secret of winter swimmers is that they not only have an adaptation to cold water, they literally thrive on it. Regular exposure to the cold, says the report, produces an enhanced tolerance of low temperatures. While mere mortals are able to increase their metabolism for a relatively short time in response to cold, winter swimmers increase their metabolism after immersion and it is still rising at the end of the swim.

One theory is that their body's protective systems respond to deep core temperatures rather than to skin temperatures, which also means they do not need to shiver to keep warm. Research also shows that there is reduced blood flow to their skin during swimming and that acts like thermal insulation: "In regular winter swimmers physiological adaptation occurs that makes them more tolerant to cold stimuli," says the report.

But the benefits don't stop there. There are, says the report, likely to be long-term beneficial health effects from regular winter swimming. There's some evidence, for example, that regular winter swimming has a beneficial effect on insulin levels which may impact on heart disease. It boosts antioxidant levels too, and higher levels of immune system cells have been found in the blood of regular winter swimmers. Other studies show that winter swimmers have 40 per cent fewer respiratory tract infections.

"Swimming is a good aerobic exercise, with proven health benefits. Swimming in cold water during the winter season is associated with significant additional physiologic alterations that could be detrimental in most individuals," says the report. "However, repeated exposure to cold stimuli results in an increased tolerance to cold, through a variety of adaptive mechanisms. A significant body of evidence raises the hypothesis that these mechanisms may also confer protection against several diseases."

Finger lengths predict disease

LOOK CLOSELY AT YOUR HANDS. Is your ring finger longer or smaller than the index, or are they about the same?

No idle question this. The answer could help you discover what diseases you are likely to get, and how long you have left.

It has been known for some time that the relative lengths of the second (index finger) and fourth (ring finger) digits differ between men and women. Men tend to have fourth digits longer than the second, while women tend to have second digits longer than fourth.

Researchers argue that such a universal feature did not evolve by chance, and that there has to be a reason why men and women tend to differ. The answer, they say, is that that the digits are markers for hormonal exposure in the womb, historical fossils of what went on in the womb in the critical first three months of life.

In particular, they are a sign of the levels of hormones that shaped the early life of the foetus when the brain, heart and other organs were growing.

A relatively long ring finger is a sign that the foetus was exposed to higher levels of the male hormone testosterone, while a relatively long index finger is a marker of oestrogen exposure. But the cocktail of hormones swilling around at the time had an effect on the whole body of the developing foetus, not just the fingers. If the ring finger is long, then all the other organs which were developing at the same time would have been exposed to higher levels of testosterone. That means, say the researchers, that the ratio of the two fingers can be used to determine the risk of disease in later life, as well as traits.

"Prenatal levels of testosterone and oestrogen have been implicated in infertility, autism, dyslexia, migraine, stammering, immune dysfunction, myocardial infarction and breast cancer. We suggest that 2D:4D ratio is predictive of these diseases and may be used in diagnosis, prognosis and in early life-style interventions which may delay the onset of disease or facilitate its early detection," say the researchers.

Other research shows that the ratio of index and ring fingers can be an indicator of sporting prowess, aggression, number of sexual partners, autism and vulnerability to depression. It has also been linked to hyperactivity.

"High testosterone before birth as indicated by digit ratio produces quite a lot of behavioural problems in terms of conduct, temper tantrums, bullying, fights with other children, hyperactivity, being easily distracted and that kind of thing. In general it applies to boys and girls. It also reduces social behaviour, the tendency not to be concerned about other children's feelings, and not being helpful if someone is hurt," says Professor John Manning, an evolutionary psychologist at the University of Central Lancashire.

For women, traits associated with having a female hand with long index finger relative to ring finger include high fertility, large family, low levels of assertiveness, being neurotic, a vulnerability to early breast cancer and low risk-taking. Women with a masculine ratio have a greater risk of low fertility, are more likely to be left-handed and are higher risk-takers, more assertive and more likely to be homosexual.

For men, traits associated with a male hand – long ring finger compared to index – include high fertility, being a fast runner and good at football, autism, low verbal fluency, aggression and good maths skills. Men with a female ratio are more likely to be good dancers, have reduced fertility, good verbal skills, poor sports skills, be poor map readers, have greater intelligence and experience more depression.

NB: Digit ratio is the length of the index finger divided by the length of the ring finger. If they are equal in length the ratio is one. If the ring finger is longer the ratio is less than one. Men in general have a longer ring finger relative to their index finger.

Arthritis is the price of having healthy ancestors

WHILE BLACK DEATH MAY HAVE GRABBED the headlines in the Middle Ages, it was the White plague – tuberculosis – that caused devastation in the nineteenth and into the twentieth centuries. One in four deaths in Western Europe and the United States were due to TB in that period, and over the last 200 years, millions of men, women and children have died from it.

With such a high attrition rate, evolutionary theory suggests that TB would have acted as a powerful genetic selective force. If a genetic mutation carries increased survival chances against TB, that gene or genes would be more likely to be passed on and to survive because those with it would be more likely to mate.

But in many cases like this future generations find that there is a cost to be paid for the survival of their ancestors. A gene that may have given some protection from the effects of cholera and diarrhoea, for example, may have led to cystic fibrosis.

In a research report, James Mobley of Pfizer Global Research and Development reports a striking link between deaths due to tuberculosis between 1780 and 1900 and cases of modern day rheumatoid arthritis.

Native Americans currently have the highest rates of arthritis worldwide, with a prevalence of 5–7 per cent. And in 1886, the TB death rate for Native Americans was around 9 per cent, the highest rate ever recorded for any population. A similar matching pattern was found elsewhere. Non-native North Americans and Western Europeans have rates of arthritis between 0.5 per cent and 1.5 per cent. The peak TB death rate in England was 1.2 per cent in 1780, and in North America, 1.6 per cent in 1800. Africa has little arthritis – less than 0.1 per cent – and medical observations throughout the nineteenth century and into the early twentieth century reported finding no cases of TB in sub-Saharan Africa.

"The epidemiology of modern-day rheumatoid arthritis is strikingly similar to the epidemiology of tuberculosis 100–200 years ago, suggesting the possibility that genetic factors that enhanced survival in tuberculosis epidemics are now influencing susceptibility to rheumatoid arthritis," he says.

But if there is a link, what could it be?

Nitric oxide is the foremost candidate because it is known to increase TB resistance. In fact, synthetic versions have been used to treat patients with the disease. It seems a reasonable hunch that anyone who had a genetic mutation that resulted in higher levels of nitric oxide might have a survival advantage in a TB epidemic. And if there is a link between TB and rheumatoid arthritis, those genes that protected against TB should be found at higher levels in arthritic patients.

That may indeed be the case. Recent advances in genetics have identified several genes linked to rheumatoid arthritis that are involved in the immune response to Mycobacterium tuberculosis infection, including TNF-a.

"The human genome undoubtedly has been shaped by our constant battle against infectious microorganisms. Random mutations that allowed our ancestors to survive epidemics and plagues have been passed down to successive generations. In most cases, there is a cost to be paid for survival through mutation," says the report. "These results suggest that rheumatoid arthritis, and possibly other autoimmune diseases, are modern-day manifestations of the genetic selective pressure exerted by tuberculosis epidemics of the recent past."

Feeling disgusted is healthy

WE'VE ALL BEEN THERE. Everyone has been disgusted at some time, and by something or other. Mouldy meat, rats, sour milk, vomit, dog faeces, creepy-crawlies and countless other stomach-churners can all trigger a feeling of disgust and nausea.

But why do we feel disgusted? If everything that has evolved and stayed with us over the last few thousands years has a use, what on earth is the purpose of feeling disgusted, and how does it work?

The answer may be quite simple. Disgust could be a primitive type of immune system that evolved in animals and now works in tandem with the much more sophisticated human system. And according to the researchers, the brain chemical serotonin could be the link.

The fine-tuned, modern human immune system is wide-ranging, intricate, highly effective and if you happen to be an alien bug, disease or virus, deadly. Its only weakness is that it has to come into direct contact with a problem before it sorts it out.

Swallow mouldy food and it will sort out the consequences, but hold a rotten bit of meat in front of your face and it can do nothing. In other words, it's reactive rather than preventive.

And that, it's suggested, is where disgust comes in. Disgust can prevent infection by stimulating avoidance, or, if it is too late, vomiting.

"We propose that there is a functional link between disgust and immunity, as both are part of a defensive continuum. Disgust acts prior to or immediately following contact with infectious threats, while immunity deals with threats that persist despite disgust reactions," say the researchers from Instituto de Ecología, Veracruz, Mexico and the London School of Hygiene and Tropical Medicine.

The suggestion is that disgust evolved first as a way of protecting animals from a variety of dangers and that it comes in two forms. Stage 1 disgust is when something potentially hazardous – like mouldy food – is spotted and avoided so that the threat does not get inside the body and cause damage. Stage 2 disgust is when the threat is inside the body before the danger is realized. In that case, disgust triggers nausea, vomiting and diarrhoea to get rid of the threat as quickly as possible.

The theory is that serotonin, the brain chemical involved in appetite and mood, plays a key role in both disgust and immune system reactions. Large quantities of the compound are also found in the tissue of gut, airways and skin, which point to its having a role in defensive reactions to external threats. The brain stem is involved in the initiation and co-ordination of nausea, and it's suggested that serotonin plays a key role in triggering vomiting.

"We propose that disgust is an evolved nervous response which motivates behaviour leading to the avoidance of infection," say the researchers. "We hypothesize that disgust acts prior to contact with the infectious agent and prevents it from getting into the body. Vomiting gets it out once inside the gastrointestinal tract, before penetration of the body boundaries."

Psychopaths are a necessary evil

MUCH OF OUR BEHAVIOUR is inherited from our parents and from previous generations. Genetic studies on twins suggest that personality traits, like neuroticism, introversions and excitement-seeking, have a substantial genetic element.

Antisocial personality disorder, which 2–3 per cent of the population have, also has a strong genetic component. But why is it still around? Many other personality traits have important and vital uses, but there is no obvious value to antisocial behaviour. So, if it is an unwanted trait, which means carriers of the genes would have been less likely to mate and pass them on, why hasn't it disappeared? After all, modern society is, for the most part, based on civilizations and people who work together and who get on, so how come the cheats survive?

"Very little has been written about one of the most fascinating aspects of the evolution of human behaviour – why has natural selection allowed antisocial personality disorder to persist given that human society is mainly co-operative and has developed through co-operation?" say researchers at the Publique Hôpitaux de Paris. The answer, it's suggested, is because they help society to be distrustful and defend itself. If there had been no villains around in their hunter-gatherer group, it's argued, our ancestors would have been too trusting and would not have survived.

The researchers present a series of arguments in support of their theory. They point out, for example, that the prevalence of the disorder means that hunter-gatherer communities of around 30 would each have had one member with antisocial tendencies.

In modern times, those with the disorder who are caught go to jail, but in earlier times exclusion from the group or death was the likely option. In Inuit society, the tradition was that a psychopath – known as *kunlangeta* – would be invited to go hunting and quietly pushed off the ice when nobody was looking.

Of course, if all the villains had been excluded or killed in this way, the genes would have been wiped out. But the researchers say that around 50 per cent of them never were detected. So the heavy cost for some was counterbalanced by the benefits the survivors gained from society, including the opportunity to mate and pass on their genes.

And what, say the researchers, would have happened if a group or a society did not contain antisocial individuals?

"Let us imagine a society or a group with all kinds of personality – except this one – which has never met a sociopath and which is not aware that this kind of behaviour exists. Such a group would probably be rapidly exploited to death," they say. "But if a group contains an antisocial personality it is forced to find weapons to use against this behaviour, to maintain watchfulness and to develop protection against these people. We can imagine that groups without antisocial individuals disappeared when they encountered these personalities because they failed to produce and to use weapons against them. In brief, antisocial personality disorder is a necessary evil."

Cystic fibrosis is a legacy of the Black Death

PLAGUE OR BLACK DEATH WIPED OUT one third of Europe's population in the Middle Ages.

An infection of rodents caused by the organism *Yersinia pestis*, it also killed more than 100 million over a 50-year period in the sixth century.

In humans, the plague can be contracted in two main ways. Bubonic plague, which has a death rate of around 70 per cent, is the result of being bitten by an infected flea, while the even more lethal pneumonic plague, with a death rate of 90 per cent, is when the infection is spread between humans by inhaling contaminated droplets in the air. There is also some evidence that it may be contracted in contaminated food.

Because of the catastrophic effects of the plague, it is possible, in evolutionary terms, that some kind of protective mechanism might have evolved among the offspring of survivors.

Such an adaptation would need to focus on at least the two main ways that the disease takes hold – through the lungs or the skin. Droplets containing the infection would need to be blocked from entering the lungs, and fleas would need to be deterred from biting the skin. As an added bonus, it should also protect the gut from infection.

So what could it be? What mechanism evolved as a way of protecting man from the plague?

According to a researcher at the Fred Hutchinson Cancer Research Center, Seattle, cystic fibrosis may be the candidate. Cystic fibrosis is a disease caused by a defective gene that is carried by millions of people. It has been estimated that as many as 1 in 10 Caucasians have the gene, but the overwhelming majority have no symptoms because in order to develop the disease, two defective genes must be inherited, one from each parent.

Around 35,000 Americans and 25,000 Europeans have the disease, and intriguingly, it occurs mostly in whites whose ancestors came from northern Europe where the plague caused the most devastation.

Once always fatal in childhood, improved treatments for cystic fibrosis have increased the average lifespan to 35 or more. Death is often the result of lung disease.

Cystic fibrosis, in theory, fits the bill as a way of protecting man from the plague. It could prevent infections getting in the lungs, it does have an effect on the skin that might deter fleas and it might have a protective effect on the gut through the pancreas.

The main symptom of the disease is the production of abnormally thick and sticky mucus which builds up in the lungs and the pancreas, and which helps in the breakdown of the food we eat. It can also affect the sweat glands and infants with the condition have salty-tasting skin, which may deter plague-carrying fleas.

"I would suggest that cystic fibrosis, the most prevalent inherited disease of people from northern European ancestry, is the result of an adaptive response to *Yersinia pestis* epidemics," says the report. "Because infection is rapidly fatal in the majority of untreated cases, a strategy of blocking the portals of entry of infection – skin, lungs, gut – is a practical way to insure survival."

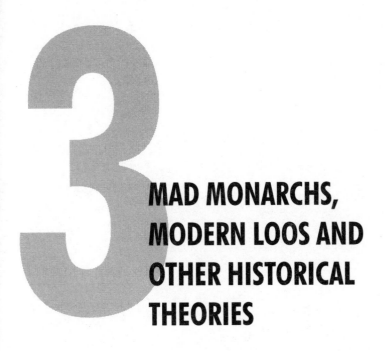

3

MAD MONARCHS, MODERN LOOS AND OTHER HISTORICAL THEORIES

Modern toilets ruin legs

HISTORY SUGGESTS THAT THE FIRST above-ground toilets appeared around 5,000 years ago.

During most of that time and through successive civilizations, the elevated seat was largely reserved for the aristocracy. Peasants continued to squat over holes in the ground.

Eventually, as time passed, everyone in the developed world moved off the ground and onto the raised seat. It was more comfortable, easier to keep clean and, when sanitation moved indoors, much more hygienic and weatherproof.

A curious, but until now little known fact is that the rise of the toilet was followed almost exactly by an increase in the incidence of leg and knee pain – sometimes, wrongly, put down to osteoarthritis – as well as leg cramps. It's estimated that 7 out of 10 people will get leg pain at some time, but in parts of the developing world, where squatting is still the norm, the incidence is much lower.

According to two American researchers, this is no coincidence. The demise of squatting and the arrival of the commode, the sit-down toilet and the chair too, mean we no longer use the muscles and joints in the way that our pain-free ancestors did. As a result, it's suggested, muscles and tendons have shortened, resulting in pain, leading to what the researchers call stiff leg syndrome.

The researchers, from Loyola University School of Medicine, have treated more than 100 patients, most of whom had knee pain and stiffness, followed by problems with the calf, hamstring and foot cramps. Around one in three had difficulty standing up from a sitting position. They were given a number of simple stretching exercises which mimic the effects of squatting.

The results show that the effects of the exercises could be immediate and dramatic. An 88-year-old man, who was referred to them after tests had failed to find the cause of dizziness and loss of balance, also had calf and hamstring cramps as well as knee pain and restless leg syndrome. Previous drug therapy had failed, but the researchers say that after 30 minutes of squat-type stretching exercises he jogged down the hospital corridor. Four months later he was still completely free of leg cramps, knee pain and stiffness, and restless legs, and was walking a mile a day.

In another case, a 62-year-old man who had been treated for 15 years for knee pain and stiffness was given a work-out programme, and after completing half an hour of stretching exercises could walk with no pain and stand up from a sitting position without using his arms.

"The major cause of leg cramps and knee pain and stiffness is inadequate muscle stretching which is a direct result of abandoning the popular practice of squatting during socialization and defecation and adopting the high sitting position on chairs and modern toilets," say the researchers. "Our toilets and our chairs are ruining our legs. Why did we ever stop squatting? Life would have been much easier sitting around eating and socializing with our buttocks close to the ground, just waddling over to the nearest hole in the ground when the need arose to defecate. Our legs were so limber and we moved with such ease."

Queen Elizabeth I was part man

DESPITE HER GOOD LOOKS, INTELLIGENCE and sparkling wit, Elizabeth I died at the age of 70 leaving no partner or heir, and ending a Tudor dynasty that had ruled England for more than a century.

Historians have speculated that she never married for psychological and emotional reasons, the result, perhaps, of a troubled childhood with her father, Henry VIII, which had left her with a deep-seated dislike of sexual intercourse. But research at Simon

Fraser University, Canada rejects these explanations as unsound and suggests that the queen was physically incapable of having a child because she had testicular feminization, a rare condition that affects 1 in 50,000 women. Also known as androgen insensitivity syndrome, the individual is genetically male, with one X and one Y chromosome, but appears to be female despite the presence of internal testes. The researchers say the external genitalia are female, but the vagina ends in a pouch or is absent, and the uterus and uterine tubes are absent or rudimentary, making childbearing impossible.

The researchers reject suggestions that Elizabeth's doctors would have known that she was infertile. That, they say, reveals an ignorance of the practice of medicine at that time, because Tudor physicians never examined the body of the patient. It is certain, they say, that Elizabeth never had a gynaecological examination of any kind.

"The diagnosis of her ability to bear children would have been made on the basis of her appearance, her behaviour, her astrological signs, and perhaps an examination of her urine and her pulse. It is possible, though unlikely, that she was questioned about her menstrual cycle, but there is no indication of this in the reports of any of her doctors," they say.

Some contemporary reports the researchers found did suggest unknown and unexplained physical defects as a reason why she remained the Virgin Queen until her death, but they have largely been rejected by historians as gossip, rumour and loose talk.

The researchers say that recent advances in the understanding of testicular feminization syndrome justify a re-evaluation of these physical defects suggested by some of Elizabeth's contemporaries.

By comparing the known symptoms of the condition and characteristics of sufferers with contemporary reports and descriptions of the queen, the researchers set out to investigate whether or not she had the syndrome and was genetically male. It's known that the condition is an inherited disorder, probably through the mother, and the paper points out that Elizabeth's mother, Anne Boleyn, had a sixth finger, a condition known as polydactylism, which has been linked to a number of other developmental disorders.

"At puberty, there is normal development of the breasts and of a female appearance. These individuals are usually pretty and attractive, above average in height, with slim hips with long extremities and large hands and feet. Their hands are often thin and elongated," they say. And that fits with contemporary descriptions of Elizabeth. Her physical appearance, personality and behaviour are all strikingly similar to the characteristics of women with testicular feminization syndrome.

Schizophrenia changed the course of English history

THE YOUNG HENRY VI (1421–71) seemed to have it all. Crowned at the tender age of 10, and described as robust, handsome and precocious, he was making decisions that affected the nation before he was 16 and negotiating peace with France at 18, while at the same time finding time to establish Eton College and King's College, Cambridge. Yet within a few years, it had all gone disastrously wrong. He was unable to rule and lost the crown in the Wars of the Roses. His wife died in poverty in exile, his only child was killed in battle and he himself was murdered, written off as a weak, inadequate and simple-minded king.

So what went wrong? How did the promising and ambitious young king become an indecisive, vindictive, witless failure, who lost everything?

According to Dr Nigel Bark from the Schizophrenia Research

Unit at the Bronx Psychiatric Center, schizophrenia is the answer. He has pieced together clues from contemporary records which suggest that the king had symptoms of schizophrenia in his twenties and thirties. Henry became indecisive in his early twenties and less involved in government. In 1447, Henry believed his uncle, Humphrey, Duke of Gloucester, was plotting to kill him and had him arrested, and at the same time he made grandiose plans for the expansion of King's College and Eton to make them bigger than all other cathedrals or colleges.

Change in personality, with evidence of paranoia, grandiosity, vindictiveness and indecisiveness or ambivalence, is not uncommon in someone developing schizophrenia, says Dr Bark. Crucially, in 1453, at the age of 31, Henry was reported to have lost his reason for a year and half and was said to be no longer capable of ruling. Reported symptoms include mutism and extreme negativity, both of which can be signs of schizophrenia. There is also some evidence he was having hallucinations.

After this major episode he was left passive and apathetic, and had lost his previous drive and interest. He was no longer active as king and when he was deposed, it was his wife Margaret, not he, who fought for the throne.

"The changes in the life of Henry VI are characteristic of schizophrenia: from precocious youth with friends and interests, ambitiously founding and designing Eton and King's Colleges, marriage and love, to increasing grandiosity, paranoia, ambivalence, and vindictiveness in his later twenties, leading to a sudden severe mental illness with withdrawal and mutism, followed by deterioration in function, apathy, and loss of interest," says Dr Bark.

"Henry's story illustrates how schizophrenia can devastate individuals and families and change the course of history. Without Henry's schizophrenia and consequent inability to rule, Edward, Duke of York would not have claimed the throne and Henry VII would have been even less likely to have. There would have been no Henry VIII or Elizabeth I."

It's possible too that there might not have been an English Reformation, nor colonial exploration and a British Empire.

Jesus, the Turin Shroud and spontaneous combustion

JAMES HAMILTON, A 71-YEAR-OLD PROFESSOR of mathematics, was standing outside his house one cold winter morning when he felt a sharp pain, not unlike a bee sting. Looking down, he saw a blue flame several inches long spouting from his leg. Alarmed, as most people would be, he tried slapping his leg to put the flame out, but failed. He then cupped his hands around the flame to starve it of oxygen, and it eventually did go out, but left a large scar.

Researchers cite the experience of the unfortunate Professor Hamilton as an example of preternatural combustion or spontaneous human combustion, a phenomenon that can produce intense and localized heat. What's more it could, it's argued, explain the marks on the Turin shroud.

"The image, of an apparently crucified corpse, on the Turin shroud is very possibly a scorch mark. Many of the reported phenomena of the shroud and of preternatural combustion do correspond," says the report.

The ancient piece of linen known as the Turin shroud is arguably the most studied artefact in human history. It appears to carry the image or outline of a crucified man, and many researchers believe it is the cloth that covered Jesus when he was placed in his tomb. The image on the cloth is said to be linked to effects of the resurrection.

The known history of the shroud itself goes back at least 600 years to northern France, although some historians say it can be traced to Constantinople where legend has it that a cloth with a miraculous image was brought to the city from Edessa in 944, only to be lost in 1204 during the fourth crusade.

The report says it's likely that the image on the shroud was produced from a heated solid object, although there is no obvious way for a cadaver to produce such a scorch mark. That, they say, is why the image has historically been put down to the effects of a supernatural event: the resurrection.

But what has been overlooked, according to the research, is that there is one natural phenomenon that could produce such a temperature — preternatural combustion of the human body when the body bursts into flames for no apparent reason.

Although the idea of spontaneous combustion is controversial and regarded by many as an urban myth, there are a number of theories that have been put forward to explain it. The so-called wick effect suggests that the clothing of the victim soaks up melted human fat and acts like the wick of a candle when it is accidentally ignited. The static electricity theory says there is a build-up of static in the body and that a spark ignites clothing which is then fuelled by melting fat. Evidence acquired from the small number of witnesses who have seen such events is that the fire usually starts as a small blue flame on the back or leg, spreading rapidly until it engulfs the whole body.

The report says that while much about preternatural combustion remains unexplained, a lot of what is known fits in with the evidence of the shroud. The obvious scorch marks, the absence of a body, traces of minerals (particularly iron and calcium) and of organic matter, plus the astonishment of those who discovered the empty tomb referred to in the New Testament all support the possibility of spontaneous combustion, it's suggested.

"For the scientist faced with two competing explanations, the one a miracle (resurrection) and the other a mystery (preternatural combustion), then the usual method is to wield Occam's razor and adopt the one involving the least unknowns as a working hypothesis," says the report.

If Jesus was consumed in such a way, the report adds, it would cast a very different light on the early history and tradition of Christianity.

Smoke made Neanderthals extinct

THE DISCOVERY MADE BY QUARRY workers in a remote cave deep in the German countryside in the summer of 1856 made history at the time and is still causing controversy today.

Their chance discovery of a skeleton as they blasted their way into a limestone cave in the little known Neander valley (Neander Tal in German) sparked a heated debate which has raged every since.

Was Neanderthal man an ancestor of modern man or a separate species, and, most intriguing of all, what happened to him? Why did he simply disappear so quickly in what was, in evolutionary terms, the blink of an eye?

Following at least 200,000 years of successful adaptation to the glacial climate of north-western Eurasia, Neanderthals disappeared between 30,000 and 40,000 years ago. They left no clues as to the cause of their demise, and that has led to many diverse theories. One suggestion is that that they came across a superior species that wiped them out; another blames climate change.

A hypothesis put forward by researchers at the National Institute of Public Health in Norway, and the University of Oslo, is that something altogether different may be to blame – cave smoke. They say that long-term exposure to smoke pollutants from fires in caves and rock shelters may have been involved in their extinction. The pollution effects may have been so great it led to genetic mutations which heralded their end.

They point out that open fires release a large amount of air pollutants, ash and smoke into the air, all of which have been implicated in short- and long-term illness, especially in children who breathe more quickly than adults and absorb much more contamination from the same volume of air. It can, they say, affect not just the eyes and skin, but also the brain, organs and the immune system in children as they develop and mature.

Dioxins are among the pollutants produced by burning wood, and 1 kg of wood produces up to 0.16 mg of dioxins, the toxic compounds which have been linked to major illness, including cancer.

A second strand of the theory uses research which has shown that smoking tobacco in early life may influence the health of succeeding generations. That, say the researchers, adds a new, multi-generational dimension to environmental effects on health.

Other research on animals shows that exposing gestating female rats to toxins resulted in a generation of offspring with increased incidence of male infertility. These defects were transferred through the male germ line to nearly all the males in the four subsequent generations.

The researchers say the ability of an environmental toxin to reprogramme the germ line and trigger a disease in later generations has significant implications for evolutionary biology, and maybe for Neanderthals too. They point out that the toxins the animals were exposed to in the experiments are similar to those produced by open fires. "A combination of epigenic modifications of DNA and other short- and long-term effects on human health by smoke might therefore have contributed to Neanderthal extinction," they say.

English Sweating Disease was really anthrax

IT IS ONE OF THE most mysterious diseases in history. The first case was reported in 1485, the last in 1551. Since then, there has not been the hint of another, and the cause is still a mystery.

In all there were five outbreaks of what was known as the English Sweating Disease and thousands died. It is thought to have been the cause of the death of Arthur Tudor, the teenage son and heir of Henry VII. Anne Boleyn too may have caught it, but survived.

Contemporary reports suggested that the disease, whose main symptoms were a high fever and extensive sweating, was highly virulent. It quickly took hold and in some cases death came in a matter of hours.

Although no one has ever tracked down the cause of the sickness, there are some clues. It affected mainly men, for example, particularly those living in rural areas. The men were always fit and healthy before they fell ill, and most of the infections seemed to occur in late summer.

Many theories have been put forward for the cause of the sickness, and most have centred on viruses of one kind or another, but over the years investigators have been unable to come up with an explanation that fits with all the evidence.

Then, in 2001, Amerithrax happened. Amerithrax is the FBI case file name for the events that occurred a week after the 9/11 terrorist attacks that destroyed the World Trade Center, when letters were sent to a number of addressees in the USA. Inside the envelopes were large amounts of spores of *Bacillus anthracis*, or anthrax. Thirteen people became ill with symptoms of inhalational anthrax and five died.

A report of the first ten cases recorded that the majority of the victims first presented with notable sweating. Patients were variously described as having night sweats, drenching sweats and profuse sweating.

Edward McSweegan from Maryland was struck by the similarity between the symptoms and those reported for the English Sweating Disease. There were other connections too. Anthrax is more common in agricultural areas, and when it does affect humans, it is mainly men, just like the Sweating Disease. The organism can live in the soil for many years, and that too fits in with the 70-year period the sweats were a problem in England.

McSweegan says that anthrax may not have been considered as a possible cause of the English Sweating Disease because documented cases of inhaled anthrax have been rare, and sweating is not a common symptom of anthrax when it is acquired through the skin or gut.

His research shows too that doctors treating the sweats in England also reported black spots on some of the victims which could have been the scabs that are often found in cases of anthrax.

His study found that most of the Sweating Disease victims were men of working age, 15 to 45. He says that wool and animal hair are common sources of anthrax spores, and that many of these men may have been associated with local wool production. Anthrax spores in contaminated wool, hair and grazing pastures can remain viable for long periods.

"Inhalational anthrax probably would have been a rare and mysterious phenomenon until widespread industrialization brought commercial wool- and hair-sorting activities indoors. The durability of anthrax spores and proximity to contaminated agricultural fields and products could have provided numerous opportunities for infection," he says.

Herrings saved us from heart disease

KNOWN AS "SILVER DARLINGS", HERRINGS were once the most widely eaten fish in Britain.

In 1913, at one port alone, Great Yarmouth, more than 1,200 million were landed by a fleet of 1,000 boats. In the same year, 5,000 million were landed at Lowestoft. But with the coming of steam drifters in around 1900, trawling for white fish became easier and they slowly replaced the herring. Within 60 years, commercial catches of herring were no longer being landed as tastes changed. Deep-sea fishing and white fish, like cod and plaice, were now in vogue, and the little oily fish that had been on the menu for more than 400 years was no longer wanted. Herring consumption went into terminal decline in Britain and many other parts of Europe where it had once been a staple.

Years after it went out of fashion and people stopped eating herring, the incidence of heart disease began to rise. In fact, figures show that as herring consumption declined, heart disease prevalence went up. Could there be a link? Had herrings been protecting people against heart disease and associated conditions?

Modern science is showing that essential fatty acids, like those found in abundance in herring and other oily fish, reduce the risk not just of heart disease and stroke, but immune and inflammatory diseases too. Millions of people now take fatty acid supplements for conditions as diverse as angina and osteoarthritis, and in countries where oily fish is still widely consumed, like Japan and Greenland, heart disease is not as prevalent.

White fish don't have the same unsaturated fatty acids, and according to this report, the decline in herring consumption means that people may have lost a natural protection against heart disease and other health problems. It says that multiple sclerosis too may be linked to a lack of fatty acids.

"In Britain, the population was quite suddenly starved of its traditional supply of oily fish at a time when new illnesses such as coronary heart disease made their appearance," it says. "The herring's oil is well recognized as having an essential fatty acid with anti-thrombotic potential and its decline may have ushered in a number of new diseases including coronary heart disease."

Gulf War Syndrome is an allergy to burgers

FOR YEARS, DOCTORS AND SCIENTISTS have been puzzling over what could possibly cause the wide range of symptoms found in many soldiers returning from the First Gulf War.

Chemical warfare agents, particularly nerve gas, as well as post-traumatic stress disorder, smoke from oil well fires, pesticides, depleted uranium weapons and exposure to solvents and corrosive liquids have all been looked at, but with no convincing links found.

So if these aren't the prime suspects, what could be responsible for Gulf War Syndrome?

According to researchers at Johns Hopkins University, an allergy to beef is to blame. It's suggested that when soldiers were immunized against various bugs and toxins before and during the conflict, they may have accidentally acquired an allergy to burgers and steaks. Beef products used in the preparation of the vaccines may have sensitized the troops to beef protein. And that explains why, when they went back home and were re-exposed to burgers, steaks and other beef products, they developed the classic symptoms of Gulf War Syndrome – fatigue, skin rash, muscle and joint pains, headache, loss of memory, shortness of breath, and stomach and breathing problems.

Gulf War Syndrome is a significant problem. A University of Chicago report, citing data from the American College of

Occupational and Environmental Medicine, says that at least 12 per cent of Gulf War veterans are currently receiving some form of disability compensation because of the syndrome.

According to the hamburger hypothesis, the immunization programme, which included a number of preparations against *Clostridium botulinus* and *Clostridium tetani* toxins, did give protection, but also triggered an allergic sensitization to other substances in the immunizing material, specifically beef protein. That arose because of calf serum, a common ingredient in solutions used to grow toxic organisms. As a result, it's suggested, some of the soldiers produced antibodies to beef, but had no allergy symptom while they were in the Gulf War zone living on beef-free rations. The allergy theory fits in neatly with the known delay in Gulf War Syndrome symptoms appearing. In many cases they did not become apparent until the soldiers returned home.

The research report also points out that beef protein tends to be stored in joint tissue, and that joint pains are among the most frequently recorded symptoms of the syndrome.

If the cause is beef allergy, then ex-soldiers with the syndrome should get relief from their symptoms by not eating beef. The report suggests they should remain on a strictly vegetarian diet for at least three or four months to make sure all the beef protein has gone. The researchers say soldiers will remain symptom-free when other meats – pork, lamb or chicken – are reintroduced into the diet, but will relapse when beef is added.

Prehistoric fires protected man from lung cancer

IT WOULD HAVE BEEN COLD, very cold. For modern man, relatively fresh out of equatorial Africa, the freezing temperatures and weather in Europe and the Arctic would have been almost unbearable.

As *Homo sapiens* expanded into northern Europe, and through the Orient to the Arctic and on to the Americas, the temperatures would have plunged even further, and the nights become a lot longer. And it got colder still when one of the largest known volcanic eruptions, the Toba eruption, reduced average global temperatures by at least 5 °C for many years. In such a hostile climate, fires would have been an almost round-the-clock necessity for warmth, cooking and protection. Keeping close to the fire could well have been the difference between life and death.

But close proximity to the fire, and especially the smoke, would have brought long-term health problems. As the population declined – and some research suggests the Toba eruption reduced the population to 10,000 breeding couples – there may have been a strong selection pressure for those who were the least sensitive to the effects of smoke to survive.

It's known that adaptation to the cold did lead to genetic changes. Northern Asians' eyelids, for example, are significantly thicker than in non-Asians, and this is thought to have evolved to protect the eyes from the wind as well as snow and ice glare.

Researchers at New York State University believe there was another adaptation – to smoke. Their theory is that progressive exposure to toxic smoke created selective pressure to develop an adaptation. In other words, a genetic variation would have evolved with the ability to tolerate smoke. If that is so, it should be possible to find evidence of increased resistance to lung disease in the descendants of those that migrated from the equator.

And some genetic research does suggest that there are differences in the susceptibility to lung cancer in ethnic groups. In order to test what they call the "fireside hypothesis", the team looked at data from the US National Cancer and the American Lung Association on the incidence and mortality of cancer of the lung, as well as trends in cigarette smoking, to see if there were any differences.

The results show significant differences in the incidence of lung cancer and death rates among different geographically descendant racial ethnic groups. For men of African descent, the odds of having lung cancer were 1.5 times higher than those of Caucasian descent, 2.14 times higher than men of Asian descent, 2.71 times higher than Alaskans or Native North Americans and 2.89 times higher than those of South American descent. The results also show that men are 2.1 times more likely than women to develop lung cancer, and 2.5 times more likely to die from it. That, say the researchers, suggests that, regardless of descent, men are more susceptible to lung cancer than females because the differences are consistent across all rates of cigarette-smoking.

The greater susceptibility of men further supports their theory, they say, because in a hunter-gatherer society, men would have spent most of the time hunting and away from the fire so there would have been less selection for a resistance to fireside smoke.

"Anthropological data coupled with data on both incidence and mortality rates due to lung cancer are consistent with the hypothesis that there may have been differential selection during human evolution for susceptibility to lung cancer among geographically separate groups, based on their reliance on fire as a source of warmth," say the researchers. "Furthermore, genetic evidence for race-specific gene mutations associated with lung disease susceptibility, along with sex differences, is also consistent with this hypothesis."

Alfred Nobel was killed by dynamite

A FEW YEARS BEFORE HIS DEATH, Alfred Nobel, the man who invented dynamite, was able to read his own obituary.

Printed in error in a French newspaper, it described the Swedish chemist, who also gave the world gelignite, as a merchant of death. "Dr Nobel, the man who became rich by finding ways to kill more people faster than before, died yesterday."

That he was wealthy is beyond doubt – his legacy still funds the Nobel Prizes – but did he pay the ultimate price for his invention? When he really did die, was he an early victim of dynamite?

Nobel is reported to have died of a stroke in Italy in 1896, but a review of the evidence by Sri Kantha suggests that years of exposure to nitroglycerine may have led to his death.

In his research, Kantha looked at evidence from personal records, including Nobel's letters and the observations of colleagues. He also analysed Nobel's work and career and matched symptoms and behaviour with new data on nitroglycerine poisoning.

There is little doubt that Nobel was exposed to nitroglycerine over a 33-year period, and that the exposure was at times intense. He worked alone, had little help and it's reported that an 18-hour working day was not uncommon. He carried out hundreds of experiments and over the years amassed a remarkable 355 patents for his work.

According to the records of Ragnar Sohlman, Nobel's assistant, Nobel's physical condition began to decline towards the end of the 1870s, and for the last 16 years of his life he suffered from deep depression and angina. He was said to catch colds very easily and was sensitive to changes in the weather. At one point he complained he was suffering from scurvy and wrote that the cure prescribed – horseradish and grape juice – was doing him no good.

In one letter he also described symptoms of migraine and

heart disease: "This letter was written when Nobel was only 54 and had eight more years to live. But the descriptions of his health problems are revealing. Repeated mention of severe migraine and angina suggests that Nobel was suffering from nitroglycerine poisoning," says Kantha.

The toxic effects of nitroglycerine have only been fully understood relatively recently. It is now known that continuous exposure to high levels of the compound can lead to heart problems by triggering spasms in key arteries. Other symptoms of nitroglycerine poisoning include headache, nausea, vomiting, abdominal cramps, convulsions, hypotension and vertigo.

"When one links the toxicological characteristics of nitroglycerine to Nobel's description of his pains, the nature of his malady becomes clear," says Kantha. "Nobel's prolonged contact with nitroglycerine in the laboratory and firing trials, lasting for over three decades, would have subjected him to long-term exposure to nitroglycerine. From his descriptions in letters about his pains, his solitary work habit and the toxic nature of nitroglycerine which came to be understood long after Nobel's death, I conclude that nitroglycerine poisoning would have been a contributing factor to his illness and premature death."

Ironically, low therapeutic levels of nitroglycerine were already being used in Nobel's time to treat angina, and it is still used today for its blood-thinning effects.

Shortly before his death, the man who converted nitroglycerine into dynamite wrote, "Isn't it the irony of fate that I have been prescribed nitroglycerine to be taken internally! They call it Trini-trin, so as not to scare the chemist and the public."

4

SEX, BLONDES AND NOISES IN THE NIGHT

Why women groan during sex

YES, YES, YES ... at last, a reason why people – especially women – groan and breathe heavily during sex.

Hyperventilation during sexual arousal can lead to a near trance-like state and that allows the less inhibited part of the brain to become more dominant. Heavy breathing also lowers blood pressure to the brain by as much as 50 per cent and alters blood levels of carbon dioxide, both of which have an effect in the brain.

"Groaning and hyperventilation are interpreted as a psycho-physiological mechanism to deepen states of sexual trance," say the researchers at the Medical School, Hanover. "Until now the implications of hyperventilation during sexual intercourse were virtually unknown."

Physical and psychological changes occur during sexual inter-course, many of them dictated by hormones. Most make an obvious contribution to the end result, the physical ability to mate, but involuntary heavy breathing when it is not physically demanded has defied explanation until now.

Short-period hyperventilation is known to induce anxiety in some people, as well as a euphoric state. Deliberate hyperventila-tion is also used to induce trance states in some African tribes. Research shows that heavy breathing can have a significant impact on the body and brain. Carbon dioxide pressure in the arteries is lowered, levels of stress and other hormones are altered and there are changes in the activity of muscles and nerves. Skin also becomes more sensitive, and the senses of touch and smell are enhanced.

The researchers say that what little work has been done sug-gests that breathing patterns change in both men and women, "but tend to be more accentuated in females which are known from anecdotal evidence to groan more and produce more sounds during sexual intercourse". Hyperventilation during sexual intercourse may intensify experiences of sexual excitement, sexual trance and orgasm.

Especially important are the different effects the changes have on key areas of the brain. Evidence from brain scans shows that oxygen consumption is mainly reduced in the neocortex grey matter and much less in the limbic structures. That, they suggest, alters the way the brain, and behaviour, is regulated. The decrease in cortical control may lead to experiences and behaviour dominated by the limbic, known as the emotional brain, which overrides inhibitions. Emotions take over, and there is a reduced ability to use cognitive mechanisms to gain control.

"This may be described as an arousal-dissociation between distinct parts of the brain which may in this case result in a more primitive mode of brain functioning," say the researchers.

The importance of being impotent

MORE AND MORE OLDER MEN are taking drugs to treat impotence, but they may be defying an evolutionary safety valve.

According to this research, impotence, or erectile dysfunction as it is now known, and decline in male fertility with age have both evolved as ways of stopping eggs being fertilized with age-damaged sperm.

Erectile dysfunction is very common in older men, and the sheer scale of the problem, and its huge impact on reproduction, means that there should, in theory, be an evolutionary explanation for it. According to the researchers, the reason older men have it is to stop them siring offspring because of the risk of passing on gene mutations in sperm which increases with man's age.

By programming impotence – a pre-planned obsolescence that kicks in when the man and his sperm reach their sell-by date – nature eliminates or substantially reduces the risk of damaged babies being born. It also avoid mothers wasting time and resources on nurturing foetuses that have a much greater risk of not surviving to term.

As Dr Ofer Gofrit, a urologist from Hadassah University Medical Centre, Jerusalem points out, survival of a species hinges on the transfer of healthy genetic material from parents to their child. If too much damaged sperm gets through, it can lead to miscarriage and a waste of resources. It may also lead to higher risk of death and of genetic mutations, both of which have resource implications for parents.

Testicular ageing and decline are thought to begin around the age of 30, with a thinning of some tissue and thickening of others, a decline in the number of sperm cells, and reduced semen volume and motility. Studies have shown a drop in the pregnancy rate of 23–38 per cent in women whose partners are aged over 50.

The report says that advanced paternal age is associated with a range of health problems, including cleft palate and many other congenital anomalies. There is a 27 per cent increase in risk of spontaneous abortion if the father is aged over 35, and a Danish study found that pregnancies fathered by a man aged 50 years or more had almost twice the risk of ending with foetal loss.

The age of the father at conception has also been linked to risk of the offspring developing schizophrenia and other mental illnesses. A Swedish study showed a 47 per cent increase in risk for each 10-year increase in paternal age, while an English study has found that some forms of leukaemia are significantly higher among children of older mothers and fathers.

To prevent or lower such risks, it's argued, nature has evolved impotence, the prevalence of which increases with age, from around 7 per cent at 18–29, to 18 per cent for men in their fifties and 76 per cent for men aged 80 and over. It has been estimated that 76.1 per cent of men aged 45 years are sexually active in contrast to only 16.7 per cent of those aged 80 years.

"The possibility of female impregnation by an elderly or sick male is realistic. This event has many potential deleterious effects. The genetic material provided by an elderly or sick male is less stable and the ability of an elderly father to support the pregnant mother and his progeny is lower. All these considerations go against the interest of the species," says Dr Gofrit. "I suggest that two complementary evolutionary mechanisms have evolved to compensate for this – decreased fertility, on the one hand, and erectile dysfunction, on the other hand. If the hypothesis is correct, then all treatments for erectile dysfunction like phosphodiesterase-5 inhibitors – Viagra and similar drugs – go against the natural Darwinian evolutionary selection process."

Sex causes high blood pressure in pregnancy

PRE-ECLAMPSIA IS SOMETHING of an enigma. Although it's a common problem, affecting more than four million pregnant women worldwide every year, its cause is unknown.

The main features are high blood pressure and a protein in the urine, and symptoms can include sudden weight gain, headaches and changes in vision.

It used to be known as toxaemia because it was thought to be caused by a toxin in the blood, but that has been shown to be wrong. Currently, there are more than a dozen potential explanations, including poor blood flow to the womb, injury to the blood vessels, an immune system problem, poor diet and a lack of various minerals.

Research at the Albert Einstein College of Medicine, New York suggests another reason – sexual activity during pregnancy and its effect on the woman's body.

The suspicions of researchers that this might be the cause were first raised by a casual observation by doctors in delivery rooms that women with the condition were usually accompanied by a man, while those without pre-eclampsia tended to have a female with them.

In a subsequent study, 72 randomly chosen teenagers were questioned about their sexual activity during pregnancy. All the 22 diagnosed with pre-eclampsia reported having sexual activity after conception – 19 throughout the pregnancy and three during the first trimester only. Thirteen patients who said they did not have sexual activity during pregnancy didn't develop pre-eclampsia. The remaining 37 patients were sexually active, but pre-eclampsia did not occur.

Just how sexual activity could cause the disease in some women is not clear. Transfer of infection and stress reaction are possibilities, but the researchers say the more probable causes are related to what's in the semen. One of the many compounds in semen is prostaglandin E2, a hormone-like substance that is known to play a part in the control of blood pressure. Another possibility is that other compounds lead to the creation of protective antibodies in the woman, which in turn impact on blood vessels and blood pressure.

The researchers say the idea suggests a rational explanation for the drop in cases of pre-eclampsia recorded in Germany during the First and Second World Wars, as well as the reported increase during the siege of Madrid. During the wars, men were absent from home, while during the Spanish siege, men and women spent more time together.

The theory may also explain why some women who do not have pre-eclampsia with a first birth nevertheless develop it with a second when they are in a different relationship. It is possible that in the first they did not have sex during pregnancy, but in the second, with a new partner, they did.

"The concept of a sexually-related origin provides possible

explanations for the lack of the disease in animals as well as for certain facts about the disease in humans," they say. "The concept would clarify the well-known fact that animals do not develop the disease spontaneously. Sexual receptivity among female animals is rigidly dependent on their hormonal status. Sexual activity during early pregnancy may conceivably induce the disease process in one of various ways. Infection and stress reaction are possibilities but the more probable causes are related to the contents of seminal fluid."

Vasectomy lowers the risk of prostate cancer

NO OTHER ORGAN CAUSES QUITE so much happiness and grief for men as the prostate gland.

In happy times, it contributes vital fluid to the semen and plays a key role in ejaculation, but in the bad times, it is affected by cancer as well as by benign disease.

Prostate cancer is the most common cancer in men in the UK and more than 30,000 new cases are diagnosed each year. Many more are undiagnosed, and the lifetime risk of a man being diagnosed with the disease is around 1 in 12.

Just what causes it is not clear, and genes, diet, age, race, lifestyle and medication have all been implicated. There is also no way of preventing it – or is there?

Research at the Institute for Research in Reproduction (ICMR), India suggests that men who have had a vasectomy may be at lower risk of prostate cancer. Their research shows that secretion of various compounds from the prostate gland is reduced after a vasectomy, suggesting that the gland may have shrunk.

Vasectomy is an important means of fertility control in men, and the operation is comparatively simple to perform. Several studies have shown that it has little effect on hormone levels or on the sex life of the man, but little work has been done on its other possible impacts.

In their study, the ICMR team compared blood levels of various compounds in 74 men who had had a vasectomy with those of fertile men of a similar age. Results show that concentrations of various compounds, including acid phosphatase, maltase, prolactin, citric acid, zinc and magnesium, which are all secreted by the gland, were much lower in the men who had undergone a vasectomy.

The researchers say that the reduction suggests that vasectomy leads to a decrease in the working of the gland and as a result, a drop in its weight and size. They suggest that after a man has a vasectomy, sperm does not enter the prostate and cannot therefore be involved in the development of any malignancy. A second benefit, they say, is that men who have had a vasectomy tend to have more sexual intercourse afterwards, and they cite research which shows that the risk of prostate cancer increases by nearly 80 per cent if semen is not ejaculated and is stored for a long period in the body.

The report says the research showed that a build-up of fluid in the prostate and an infection could lead to sperm entering the prostate cells and triggering malignant changes, something that would not happen after a vasectomy.

"We propose that vasectomy may lead to decrease in the incidence of prostatic tumours," they say. "It may reduce the probability because, after vasectomy, the entry of sperms into the prostate is automatically stopped. In addition, after vasectomy, frequency of intercourse may be increased due to the reduced fear of pregnancy. This increase in the frequency of sexual activity may result in reducing the prostatic residue or secretions."

A cure for infatuation

FOR THOUSANDS OF YEARS, the hunt has been on for libido-boosters and aphrodisiacs that increase sexual desire and performance. And over the years almost everything has been tried – from dried beetles, chilli and oysters, to ground deer antlers and the sexual organs of a tiger. Each has its devotees – Casanova is reputed to have put at least some of his success down to eating several oysters for breakfast – and some research suggests there may be a grain of truth in a few of them.

But while poets, philosophers and scientists have looked for the chemistry behind falling in love, no one, at least until now, has looked at the idea of an antidote, a cure for infatuation and love sickness.

According to researchers at the University of Alabama and Tabriz Medical University, Iran, a couple of hormones – melatonin and vasotocin – might be just what the lovesick need.

Intense romantic love is a universal phenomenon, a complex mix of erotic and emotional components. What is known is that in its early stages it is associated with specific physiological, psychological and behaviour changes, including euphoria, obsessiveness, intense, focused attention on a loved one and a craving for emotional and physical closeness with the target of the affection.

Some researchers believe such love is a specific emotion separate from the physical sex drive and more difficult to control. It is also thought that it works through areas of the brain associated with the reward system, and that the brain chemical dopamine is heavily involved. Key to it all, say the researchers, is the pea-sized pineal gland near the centre of the brain which produces melatonin. This is involved in the regulation of the day/night cycle and is produced at night, but inhibited by light, and plays a big part in the circadian cycle.

But it may have other effects. The researchers say that melatonin has also shown anti-dopamine activities in part of the brain, while a second hormone produced by the pineal gland, arginine-vasotocin, has been found to play a key role in romantic love.

In their report "A cure for infatuation? The potential 'therapeutic' role of pineal gland products", the authors suggest that giving the two hormones may be a cure for unrequited love.

"We hypothesize that the pineal gland hormones may attenuate the romantic love, particularly in its early stages, through their anti-dopaminergic properties and inhibitory effects on the caudate nucleus, which is a crucial brain region in the evolution of love," they say. "Hence, exogenous administration of the melatonin and vasotocin might be a potential therapeutic option in attenuating intense romantic love."

Winter depression stops sex

THERE MAY BE MORE to winter depression than meets the eye.

It had been thought that seasonal affective disorder, or SAD, was simply a response to the cold temperature and the long dark nights of winter. And it's true that the prevalence of the condition, with its classic symptoms of low mood, lethargy, social withdrawal, decreased libido and increased appetite and weight gain, goes up as distance from the equator increases.

Seasonal mood changes have been reported for thousands of years, and while symptoms of SAD are almost certainly triggered by lack of light, the unsolved question is why millions suffer. Could it be that there was, at least until relatively recently, an evolutionary advantage to what is now seen as a disease?

According to a researcher at the Royal Cornhill Hospital, Aberdeen, winter depression may have been a way of discouraging sex and conception so that babies would be born at the healthiest time of the year, between late winter and early summer.

In the old days of the hunter-gatherer, a baby born when food supplies were likely to be more plentiful, temperatures warmer and days longer would have had much better survival chances. Conception in winter, on the other hand, would have led to an autumn birth, with falling temperatures, nights drawing in and limited food supplies over the critical months ahead.

The optimum time to be born – between February and June in the northern hemisphere – requires conception between May and September. That is the time when SAD sufferers are at their most active, with increased mood and heightened libido. The peak times for SAD are the six months of autumn and winter, when conceptions need to be avoided in order to maximize survival chances.

"Recurrent winter depression/attenuated hibernation, it is hypothesized, both encouraged pregnancies at the most advantageous time of the year and discouraged them at disadvantageous times," says the report. "Lower energy, social withdrawal, decreased mood and lowered libido are factors which would discourage both sexes from seeking a mate and, if they found a potential mate, that mate would be less attractive to them."

The report also points out that while SAD does occur in men, it is mostly women in their reproductive years who report symptoms. Another piece of evidence is that while the incidence of SAD does increase with distance from the equator, in genetically stable areas, like Iceland, the incidence is relatively low. That could be because the lack of sex and mating in SAD people would have meant they would be less likely to have offspring to pass on their genes and their numbers would therefore have declined.

The report says the evidence shows that at temperate latitudes, recurrent winter depression was a genetically transmitted adaptive mechanism which improved the likelihood of reproductive success for the hunter-gatherers.

Now, of course, it is no longer an advantage. With modern indoor working and ample food supplies, and warmth and light, survival chances for babies are pretty much the same all year around. As a result winter depression is now seen as a disorder. Indeed, studies of populations at higher latitudes who are geographically immobile suggest that recurrent winter depression may constitute a reproductive disadvantage. If so, says the report, it should become less common over the next several thousand years.

Gentlemen prefer blondes

WHAT'S SO SPECIAL ABOUT BLONDES? Why is it that many men, and especially older men, are attracted to fair looks and locks? Why do blondes seem to have all the fun?

Many explanations have been put forward. It's been suggested that men prefer rounder faces and that blonde hair is kinder to the outline of the face. It's also been proposed that blondes have softer, childlike skin, which men find attractive, or that they evolved as a genetic mutation 10,000 or so years ago which men have evolved to value because of its original scarcity.

According to research from the Brain & Perception Laboratory at the University of California at San Diego, they are all off the mark. The answer is that blonde hair, like the peacock's tail or the rooster's bright-red plumage, is a sign of fitness.

The evolutionary reason why men are attracted to blondes is that the hair and skin colour make it easier to spot problems. The researchers point out that anaemia, cyanosis (a sign of heart disease), jaundice and skin infection are all much easier to detect in fair-skinned individuals than in brunettes.

The theory is that in ancestral times, when bugs and infections were thick on the ground, there was an evolutionary need to be attracted to a healthy mate to increase the chances of fertility, pregnancy and the birth of a healthy child. Hence blondes became man's first choice for mating.

A second theory behind the preference for blondes is that they have reduced protection from ultraviolet radiation which causes their skin to age faster than brunettes'. As a result, visible signs of ageing – age spots and wrinkles – are usually easier to detect in blondes, so men find it much easier to judge their age. Since fertility in women declines rapidly with age, and ageing men prefer young women as sexual partners, it's suggested that blondes might be preferred because the signs of ageing are easier to detect in them.

It's also possible that some visible signs of attraction or sexual interest, including blushing, are easier to detect in blondes. As a result, the likelihood that courtship gestures will be reciprocated and consummated can be predicted with greater confidence in a blonde.

"In summary, I suggest that gentlemen prefer blondes in order to enable them to detect the early signs of parasitic infestation and ageing – both of which indirectly reduce fertility and offspring viability," says the report.

House smells turn teenage girls into women

OVER THE LAST CENTURY THERE has been big drop in the age of menarche among women in most industrialized countries. For most girls in Victorian England, menarche came at the age of 14, but by the 1940s, it had reduced to 12.8. Research from the USA shows that for girls born in the 1980s it is now 12.2 years, and dropping at the rate of about one month a decade.

The onset of menarche is an important physical and mental milestone for girls, and there have been a number of attempts to explain the decline in age, including better health and nutrition, and other environmental factors. But according to research at Rutgers University, there is an alternative explanation: the impact that social changes have had on the home. With mothers spending more time out of the home at work and fathers spending less time at work, the cocktail of human body smells in the home has changed.

At the centre of the theory are pheromones, chemicals that transmit unconscious messages to members of the same species, Much research has been done on animals, which have a more developed sense of smell, but an increasing body of research is showing they can have an effect on humans too.

One study found that within a few months of living together in close proximity, women synchronize their menstrual cycles. It also found that exposure to males affects the length of the menstrual cycle, and that women with little contact with males had longer menstrual intervals than females who had three or more interactions with men a week.

The Rutgers researchers point out that as the age of menarche has dropped over the last 150 years, there have also been big social changes. The industrial revolution and more recent labour changes and equality laws mean that there has been a significant increase in the numbers of women working away from the home. The percentage of the US female population employed outside the home went up from 18 per cent in 1890 to 45 per cent in 1974.

Unemployment and changes in working practices, and the decline of labour-intensive heavy industries, have also led to reduced working hours for men, allowing them to spend much more time at home. The more recent trend for men to work at home has further increased the time they can spend with their family.

Family size has also decreased. For mothers born between 1881 and 1885, 33 per cent were in families of seven or more children, whereas only 10 per cent of their daughters had families of this size.

The researchers say that all those social changes have resulted in pre-pubertal girls having reduced exposure to their mothers, whose pheromones have a delaying effect on menarche, and more exposure to their fathers, which leads to earlier menarche. There is also reduced exposure to older female siblings who are now more likely to go out, either to school or work.

"We suggest that pheromones play a role in determining age of menarche, and changes in pheromonal exposure have influenced the trend," say the researchers. "We suggest that with the advent of social change (industrial revolution, mothers working away from the home, shorter work week, smaller families with few older siblings), young females are exposed to fewer inhibitory pheromones from adult females, and more stimulatory pheromones from adult males."

Baby blues are caused by lack of sex

FORGET ABOUT PILLS, POTIONS and psychotherapy, it's sex that can beat the blues.

When a woman has sexual intercourse with her partner, she gets not just love, but a mix of hormones and other substances in the seminal fluid that can have a powerful effect on her brain chemicals and improve mood. But after giving birth, there may be a disinterest in sex for some weeks, leading to a drop in concentrations of the compounds, resulting in postnatal depression.

According to a researcher at Otago University, New Zealand, seminal secretions include oestrogens, testosterone and at least 13 prostaglandins (hormone-like substances that have an effect on neurotransmitters in the brain).

Interestingly, evening primrose oil, widely used to treat symptoms of premenstrual tension, including depression, has high levels of the omega 6 fatty acid gammalinolenic acid, which is converted by the body to prostaglandin E1. In one study, evening primrose oil was associated with a 74 per cent drop in depression symptoms. Other research has found that patients with depression have significantly less prostaglandin in their blood than healthy patients.

The Otago University report says the vagina is able to absorb the hormones and other compounds from seminal fluid. Small ridges in the tissue make the surface of the vagina well suited for absorbing fluids, and this hormonal cocktail may eventually end up in the blood and on its way to the brain. Animal studies have shown that levels of hormones can be increased 21-fold through vaginal tissue.

According to the report, one reason why women may have reduced levels of prostaglandins after giving birth is that their natural levels of essential fatty acids, compounds that are turned into prostaglandins, have been reduced as a result of the pregnancy. But another theory is that the woman is not getting any prostaglandins from her partner. Research suggests that intercourse does not usually happen for around 4–6 weeks after the woman gives birth. As a result, it's suggested, there is a decline in the prostaglandins being absorbed by the vagina which would add to the decline in the mother's mood.

To support the case, the report details the case of a woman treated for depression and other symptoms. She was first given essential fatty acids to make up for the lack of hormones that she normally would have obtained from her husband. As a result, says the report, there was an improvement in her mood, a change in her sexual behaviour and a resumption of the couple's usual sexual activity.

"Because the hormones found in seminal fluid are absorbed in significant amounts, there is likely to be an effect on the thinking, mood and behaviour of women," says the report. "If these observations and deductions are correct, regular amounts of seminal plasma may be important in maintaining a woman's affective health." It adds, "While the general ethos in many Western societies is critical of men, particularly because of their sexuality, this hypothesis, if corroborated, would place a some-what greater value on men and their sexual activity."

Gum disease causes small babies

IT'S KNOWN AS THE MEXICAN paradox and it has baffled doctors for years. Mexican-American women have a similar low socio-economic status as non-Hispanic Blacks, but they have a much lower rate of low birthweight births. Birthweight is often lower in less affluent classes, but the Mexican rates were not just a little higher, despite the same levels of poverty as non-Hispanic Blacks, they were approaching those of more affluent American whites. Research, based on 1.6 million births, shows that the rate of low birthweight (under 2 kg) was 5.7 per cent among white infants, and 5.2 per cent among Mexican-Americans, but 12.5 per cent among non-Hispanic Black infants.

The same paradox has been seen in other parts of the world, and the reasons remain far from clear.

To investigate, researchers at Tulane, Louisiana State and East Tennessee State Universities analysed national health data for the USA for other variables among the three groups. What they found was that the rates of gum disease in the three were pretty much in line with the low birthweight rates. Almost a third of non-Hispanic Black pregnant women had periodontal disease, compared to 20 per cent of Mexican-Americans and 10.7 per cent of non-Hispanic Whites. In other words, the risk of having gum disease was 50 per cent lower in Mexican-American women compared to non-Hispanic Black women.

Gum disease, which affects more than half the adult popula-tion, usually begins with a build-up of plaque, a sticky coating made up of food and bacteria, which leads to inflammation of the gums, bleeding and gingivitis. If this early-stage disease is not treated it can develop into periodontitis where the gums swell, forming pockets around the teeth in which plaque collects. In the severe form, found in up to 20 per cent of people, it triggers chronic inflammation and immune reactions resulting in a shrinking of the gum, bone and soft tissues supporting the teeth. Eventually, teeth can become loose and may have to be removed.

Gum disease, especially periodontitis, has been linked to a range of other conditions as diverse as atherosclerosis, premature birth, higher sugar levels, diabetes, immune problems, anaemia, respiratory disease, liver and cholesterol problems, and rheumatoid arthritis. There's some suggestion that it may also help explain some of the link between depression and heart disease.

Many of these diseases involve inflammation, and one theory is that compounds associated with inflammation that trigger gum disease have an adverse effect on other organs and tissue. Dentists who extracted teeth from around 70 patients with advanced gum disease found that there was a big drop in blood levels of compounds associated with heart disease risk.

The Tulane-led researchers suggest that periodontal disease may trigger an inflammatory response that puts compounds in the blood throughout the body which lead to a number of problems in pregnancy, including premature delivery and low birthweight.

"Because periodontal disease could lead to an increased risk of preterm birth and low birthweight and because the prevalence of periodontal disease is relatively low in Mexican-American women during and outside pregnancy, we speculate that this lower prevalence may explain, at least partially, the lower rate of low birthweight and preterm birth in Mexican-American women," say the researchers. "Our hypothesis is that the paradox of lower rates of low birthweight and preterm birth in Mexican-American women may be explained by the lower prevalence of periodontal disease in this population before and during pregnancy."

Condoms increase the risk of breast cancer

WHEN RESEARCHERS COMPARED MORE THAN 300 women with and without breast cancer, they found a curious link between condom use and the incidence of the disease. The results showed that women who had used barrier forms of contraception in their early reproductive lives were five times more likely to develop breast cancer.

According to Arne Gjorgov of the University of Pennsylvania School of Medicine, not using barrier methods could halve the incidence of the disease. "The risk of developing breast cancer is about five times greater in women who use barrier methods than in women who use non-barrier contraceptive methods," he says. "The reduction of the incidence of breast cancer by eliminating the barrier contraceptive techniques would be not less than 50 per cent in married women in the population."

The theory is based on evidence that certain hormonal compounds found in semen, including prostaglandins, are biologically active. Prostaglandins work in a number of ways, including regulation of inflammation, and synthetic versions are used to induce childbirth. In barrier contraception, the woman is not exposed to semen, so any protective effect there might be would be lost.

To test the theory, women were asked a number of questions, including the methods of contraception they used from puberty until the age of 40. Barrier contraceptive methods were classed as including condom, withdrawal, long-term abstinence and celibacy. Non-barrier contraceptive methods were diaphragm, pill, IUDs, rhythm, foam, jelly, douche and female sterilization.

The results show that women who were not exposed to semen in their early productive life, either through barrier contraception or male partner infertility, were 4–5 times more likely to develop breast cancer. "The relative risk is a result which may suggest that barrier contraception as well as the male infertility play more than a chance role in this malignant disease in married women," says the report.

It is possible that male partner infertility might have skewed the results — it could be a marker for older age in the women, for example — but when contraceptive methods alone were taken into account, the relative risk actually went up to 5.3 times.

5

IT'S THE SUN (AND MOON) WHAT DONE IT

Sunny days make men violent

BEWARE OF NATIONAL LEADERS and violent men in the summer. Watch out especially in August, the peak month of the year for starting wars, invasions and other acts of hostility, as well as for individual acts of aggression, from assault and rape, to aggravated burglaries.

The reason? It could, say researchers, be down to day length and its effects on brain chemicals like serotonin, which is involved in mood regulation and which is also the compound that is therapeutically manipulated by the world's most popular family of antidepressants.

It's long been suggested that the length of the day, the so-called photoperiod, can have an effect on a number of conditions, including mania and depression, as well as suicide and admissions to mental hospitals. Generally, the less light, the greater the prevalence of these disorders. Research in Scandinavia, for example, has shown that rates of depression are much higher in the long winter months, and other work had shown serotonin to be implicated.

But could the length of day and its impact on brain chemistry have a much wider effect, one that goes beyond depression? Is it possible that a lot of light makes people more violent?

A team from Ben Gurion University, Israel analysed data from four continents in their search for evidence of such a link. They reviewed data on violent and non-violent crimes, and historical records for the starting dates of more than 3,000 wars or acts of hostility. They reasoned that although violence by individuals and states starts for a wide range of economic, religious, nationalist and other reasons, aggression may play a part in the final decision and timing of the start of hostilities.

Results for individual violent offences did show a pronounced annual pattern. In the northern hemisphere, violent crime peaked in July and August and was at its lowest in December–February. In the southern hemisphere, the reverse was found – a peak in December–January and a low point in June–July.

They found that violent crimes occurred 2–3 times more frequently during the two summer months in both hemispheres. In contrast, non-violent offences were distributed equally throughout the year and showed no seasonal rhythm or link with photoperiod.

When the team looked at the timing of the outbreaks of wars, a similar pattern was found. In the northern hemisphere, there was a peak in August and a trough in December and January.

"The annual rhythms in the acts of aggression, both in the northern and the southern hemispheres, have a statistically significant positive correlation with the annual rhythm of the photoperiod duration in the same geographical regions," say the researchers, who suggest that their findings have important practical implications for crime prevention, law enforcement and war prevention. They say the brain chemical mechanism that could be at work is not known, but that it is probably the same for individual and collective aggression.

The prime suspect is serotonin. The suprachiasmatic nucleus, a critical brain structure involved in the circadian cycle, has a lot of serotonin nerve cells, and the researchers say many animal studies show a link between increased aggression and low levels of serotonin.

Research on humans has come to similar conclusions. Aggressive soldiers tend to have lower levels of the chemical; so do murderers and suicides.

"Thus we hypothesize that seasonal changes, influenced by changes in the duration of the daily photoperiod, in brain levels of serotonin in affective patients – who have an already disrupted serotonergic function – and in aggressive people, as well as those with affective personalities, leads to seasonal affective episodes manifested by individual violent crime and collective acts of hostility," they say.

The sun causes schizophrenia

DESPITE BEING KNOWN TO BE a distinct mental health disorder for more than a century and much investigated, schizophrenia remains a puzzle. Its cause is still not known, and while genes are thought to play a role, many other possibilities have been investigated, including viruses, stress, drugs and childhood deprivation.

It's a disease that also has some curious epidemiological features. Scientists have for example found geographic differences as well as a link between the date of birth and risk. In the northern hemisphere, people with schizophrenia are more likely to be born in February and March, and a lack of sunshine with consequent low levels of vitamin D affecting the developing of the child's brain has been blamed.

Another theory also points at the sun, but not at the ultraviolet radiation or vitamin D, but at sunspots on the sun itself. The theory is that the sunspots have an impact on the developing brain, possibly, it's suggested, through a sudden, invisible, dramatic magnetic storm that engulfs the earth.

It may seem unlikely that a largely unseen and unnoticed event so far away could impinge so dramatically on life and health on earth, but other research has suggested otherwise. Some studies have found links between sunspot activity and flu epidemics, as well as birth rates, epileptic seizure frequency, hip breakages in older women, immune activity, disruptive social behaviour and lifespan. At least one study has shown that hospital admissions for mental disorder rise during sunspot activity, while another points to a worsening of symptoms in some mental illness patients.

According to the report, sunspots are relatively cool regions that appear as dark spots on the surface of the sun, which can last for several days and which have magnetic fields thousands of times stronger than the earth's own magnetic field.

Trying to find a link with events millions of miles away in space is not as difficult as it may seem. Citing research on other sunspot–health links, the report says the evidence points to microwaves, and microwave radiation from the sun increases several thousand-fold during solar spot and flare activity. Such waves, it's suggested, have been shown to increase cortisol and stress levels in animals, and the area of the human brain that deals with stress is also suspected to be involved in schizophrenia.

One possibility is that sunspot activity leads to a fall in foetal levels of zinc which may result in damage to brain tissue, which has a high zinc requirement. Those who are genetically vulnerable to developing the disease would then be at a higher risk. "This paper suggests that schizophrenia is caused by some factor associated with sunspots," says the report.

But if the sunspots do lead to the disease, why, asks the report, are there no cases of the disease recorded much before 1800? According to the report, a radiocarbon dating study has shown that in the period 1000–1715 there was a total sunspot absence separated by short periods when sunspot number never rose above 50. This, it says, would explain why there are no case descriptions of schizophrenia in the medical literature before 1800 and a continuous increase in incidence from that date.

The sun fixes lifespan

THE FUTURE REALLY MAY BE mapped out in the heavens.

Birth dates and the position of the sun do have an effect on health, wealth and happiness, as well as longevity, mood and creativity, according to new research. But it has little or nothing to do with astrology. Life on earth and longevity are influenced not so much by Taurus, Aries and the other birth signs, but by where and when you are born, or more precisely, the latitude of birth and the prevailing solar radiation.

Being born on the critical latitude 53 N, which runs through northern England, taking in Liverpool, increases the likelihood of being creative, but it is also where male foetuses have the lowest chances of survival. Those born on this latitude are also more likely to be mathematicians.

According to the research, latitude is a marker for length of day, levels of light exposure and ultraviolet radiation which can have a good or bad effect on the developing foetus.

There are number of theories, both environmental and genetic, as to why there should be geographic differences in prevalence of disease, but new research suggests that ultraviolet radiation is the culprit. The theory is that the levels of radiation influence embryonic tissues through DNA mutation and also predispose or protect against various diseases later in life.

"It is intriguing to find that where and when we are born does have an influence on our futures. This is not astrology, this is based on basic science. But if you think about it, it's not hard to believe. The sun has been around for a few billion years, so it would be very surprising if life did not march to the beat of the sun, and of course it does. We adapt to it, and we are stressed by it. Ninety-eight per cent of the time it is benevolent, but one or two per cent of the time it is destructive," says Dr George Davis, an American physician and scientist who led the research.

"We have found evidence that latitude, or variation in light, is an added stress to the immune system, especially at 53–54 N latitude, which is involved in nearly all human disease. We believe that solar cycle radiation has been a fundamental engine of evolution, forcing organisms to adapt to mutagenic UVR and producing enough damage to instigate genetic variation."

The ultraviolet radiation theory that light exposure has an effect on the immune system has been tested in a study of the prevalence of 37 types of disease among more than 250,000 people in Maine. The birth dates of all the men and women were compared with levels of solar activity around that time. The results show that in each of the years that peak solar radiation was recorded there was an overall increase of 28 per cent in disease for people born in those years. "It appears unlikely that there would be only a chance association without causality for such a wide spectrum of diseases in so many persons over seven solar cycles. We propose that solar radiation peaks are the prime cause for genetic disruption of all life," say the researchers.

Ultraviolet radiation may also alter brain chemistry early in embryo development, and they cite research showing that most of the world's greatest mathematicians over several centuries were more often than not conceived near the summer solstice. Knowing the birthplaces of the majority of these great mathematicians over the last 400 years, the researchers have calculated that 54 per cent were born at a latitude of 53 N.

"We believe that UVR intensity and variation are at the highest at 54 latitude, and that this latitude might present a greater stress and greater risk of disease. At the same, there is a trade-off in that there is in increase in creativity," says Dr Davis.

Work by the same research group at Psybernetics Inc., Maine suggests that every decade or so the sun throws out more ultraviolet than usual, resulting in additional and excessive DNA damage to human beings. The result, they say, is that maximum lifespan will stay at about 100.

"We present evidence that the sun determines the limits of longevity for the longest-living complex organisms. Although solar cycles occur every eight to 14 years, we show that 28 per cent of these cycles irregularly release up to 300 per cent more ultraviolet radiation than usual," says Dr Davis. These bursts of radiation, it is suggested, damage our DNA, which over time reduces our ability to fight disease. Our bodies can take only about 100 years' worth of these regular UV batterings before we ultimately succumb.

Flu epidemics are affected by the sun

FOR CENTURIES, ASTRONOMERS PUZZLED OVER the meaning of sunspots. First recorded in ancient China around 2,000 years ago, their existence was later confirmed by Galileo and his contemporaries with their new telescopes, shortly before they ran into trouble with the Vatican for suggesting that the heavens were not perfect and that the sun rather than the earth was the centre of the solar system.

It's now known that sunspots, small dark patches that appear on the surface of the sun, are cooler and darker than the surrounding material. But although they are cooler, the sun overall heats up when they appear.

Magnetic activity that accompanies the sunspots can result in big changes in ultraviolet and x-ray radiation levels, which can cause the earth's atmosphere to heat up and expand, and increase ozone levels. Some researchers believe that a long period of solar inactivity may cause colder temperatures on earth and be responsible for the Little Ice Age of 1645–1715.

If sunspots can have such a profound effect on the earth's temperature, could there be other, as yet undiscovered effects? Could sunspots be linked to pandemic flu?

According to research at the Chinese University of Hong Kong, sunspots not only explain the timing of major flu outbreaks over the last 300 years, they can be used to predict when the next one will occur. And it is going to be between 2008 and 2013.

The theory is that sunspots affect the climate, which in turn affects the behaviour and activity of migratory birds that carry and spread the flu virus.

Pandemics can have catastrophic effects – the 1918 Spanish flu killed more Americans than all the wars of the twentieth century – and they occur when there is a sudden change in the virus that results in a new influenza A subtype. That new virus can be the result of a virus mixing effect in animals, and the last two pandemic viruses are thought to have been combinations of bird and human influenza viruses. When that kind of sudden, dramatic antigenic shift happens, most people have little or no protection against the new virus.

Wild birds are reservoirs of the flu virus, and their migratory behaviour, which affects the speed at which the virus is spread globally, is affected by climate. The Hong Kong researchers say there is mounting evidence that solar activity has an influence on terrestrial climate, and that the migration pattern of some birds is affected by sunspot cycles. Other research has shown that the arrival dates of some migratory birds, including cuckoos, larks and swallows, are delayed when there are increased numbers of sunspots.

It is suggested that viruses are spread to other animals through contamination of water in the farms along the flight paths of migratory birds. Changes in climate could also tend to increase contacts between animals which would also increase the risk of a new virus being created.

To test the theory, the researchers looked at flu pandemics between 1700 and 2000 and found that there was a link with the number of sunspots – the greater the number of sunspots, the bigger the risk.

"Sunspot cycles may be an inexpensive and easy method to detect influenza pandemics. The next high-risk period will be around 2008–2013 and it may suggest we be more alert and be prepared in order to minimize unnecessary deaths as a result of influenza," they say.

Gout attacks are caused by the moon

OVER THE CENTURIES, MUCH HAS been blamed on the moon, from mental illness to changes in fertility. But no one has sought an extraterrestrial explanation for an attack of gout until now. According to this theory, the frequency of gout attacks varies with the phases of the lunar cycle and may be due to the gravitational pull of the moon and its effect on those painful sharp crystals in swollen and throbbing big toes.

Gout is caused by the build-up of uric acid which results from the breakdown of compounds called purines found in all body tissue and in many foods, including liver, dried beans and peas. Normally the acid passes through the kidneys and out of the body in urine, but it can build up in the blood when there is too much. The acid then circulates in the blood and gets into joints, most commonly the big toe, where it forms crystals and causes acute inflammation and pain.

In many cases, the gout flares up for no apparent reason, and in the study at the Research Institute of Rheumatic Diseases, Slovakia the scientists looked at whether or not the moon had a role to play. They reviewed a number of attacks reported by patients to see if there were any trends that suggested a link with the lunar cycle.

The results show that there was indeed a lunar effect, with the biggest peaks happening under the new and full moon, coinciding with the peak tidal effects of the moon.

"Lunar effects on life and man are usually discussed with scepticism often rightly, due to inappropriate statistical treatment of the underlying data. There is according to our knowledge no report about gout and the moon at all," say the researchers. The scientists, who say they have found a similar lunar pattern with bronchial asthma attacks in children, say the big challenge is how to explain a mechanism by which the moon could have such a profound effect.

One theory is that melatonin, the hormone which plays a key role in orchestrating many functions, and whose production is linked to light and dark, could be implicated. Another suggestion is that the moon may have an effect on the crystals themselves. The theory is that the peaking of gout attacks around the new and full moon could be down to a slight gravitational pull of the moon on the crystals.

Around the times of a full and new moon, it seems, it may be best to keep the painkillers handy.

Chest pains are caused by the moon

SPONTANEOUS PNEUMOTHORAX IS A COLLECTION of air or gas in the chest, which can causes the lung to collapse. It most often occurs in tall, thin men between the ages of 20 and 40 and is usually caused by the rupture of a small air – or fluid-filled sac in the lung called a bulla.

Although it can be associated with disease, including asthma or cystic fibrosis, in many cases there is no apparent reason for the condition, whose symptoms include chest pain, shortness of breath and cough.

A number of potential causes have been suggested, including pressure changes triggered by the weather, particularly thunderstorms, and the effects that they have on the sacs in the lungs. When pressure increases, it's been argued, sacs are more likely to rupture.

To try to find a better answer, doctors at the Institute of Preventive and Clinical Medicine, Bratislava, set out to see if they could come up with any clues using information taken from a patient survey. They reviewed the cases of 203 men and 41 women, almost half of them under 30, whom they had treated for the condition.

They found that there did appear to be a pattern to the admissions, and that the timing and frequency did not seem to be random, but operated over a two-week cycle. In fact, when they analysed the data, there were two distinct peaks for both men and women. One came exactly one week before the new moon, and the second one week after.

Just how the moon could have such an effect is not clear, but the researchers say it might exert an influence through gravitation in much the same way that it affects the tides on earth. Slight pressure changes at certain times of the lunar cycle, it's suggested, may be enough to trigger the rupturing of a sac.

Such a lunar effect could, it's argued, affect fluid balances in the small airways of the respiratory system which can cause airway obstruction, leading to a rupture of the sacs in the lungs.

"To our knowledge, an association between a specific moon phase and the development of spontaneous pneumothorax has not been considered so far. The moon with its phases might exert an influence on man by gravitation, as it affects the tide," say the researchers. "The most outstanding finding is the peak located one week before the new moon. The second highest peak in that one week after the new moon. Further studies and new statistical observations are needed to challenge the statement that lunar phenomena are an artefact of romance or just a myth."

How weather affects mood

FOR YEARS, RESEARCHERS HAVE PUZZLED over how the weather could affect mood and behaviour.

Why is that people are more depressed at night or in the winter? Why are they happier when it's sunny and more miserable when it's raining? Why do impending thunderstorms cause depression and, most intriguing, what causes the changes in mood and behaviour up to three days before the start of the *sharav* wind in Israel?

Changes in light, dark and temperature have all been implicated, but what's the mechanism?

According to researchers at Hillside Hospital, New York, it may be all down to changes in atmospheric electricity which affects the body's acupuncture points, which in turn has an impact on levels of brain chemicals involved in mood.

One of the most popular forms of complementary medicine, acupuncture involves sticking needles into specific points of the skin with the aim of easing symptoms of a wide range of conditions, from neck pain and osteoarthritis, to dental pain and bedwetting.

There is increasing evidence that acupuncture works, and the traditional theory is that it regulates the flow of vital energy, *Qi*, that circulates through a series of invisible channels in the body to remove blockages, boost energy flow and trigger healing. More modern interpretations are that the needles trigger the release of endorphins, the feel-good chemicals, or that they interfere with the pain receptors or stimulate the nervous system. One of the newest versions of the therapy is electro-acupuncture where the points are stimulated not by fine needles but by a pulsating electrical current.

So, if acupuncture points can be worked with an electrical device, they could, at least in theory, respond to significant changes in atmospheric electricity. According to the researchers, the effect of atmospheric electricity does resemble that of acupuncture. In fact, they say, acupuncture needles can be considered as a kind of antenna or aerial.

It's argued that when the points respond to stimulation triggered by specific weather conditions, moods can change. The researchers point out that animal studies have shown that both acupuncture and electro-acupuncture can stimulate the release of norepinephrine and serotonin, brain chemicals that are involved in mood.

"Acupuncture-like effects of atmospheric electricity cause changes in brain neurotransmitters which affect mood and behaviour," say the researchers. "This change causes alterations in the functioning of neurotransmitters in the central nervous system, which leads to a shift in the psychological condition."

Why Greenlanders have less cancer

ONE OF THE MANY UNEXPLAINED features of cancer is the widespread geographical variations in the prevalence of the disease. Some areas of the world have vastly greater incidences of disease than others. In parts of China, for example, the incidence of prostate cancer is 500 times less than it is in the USA, which has double the rate found in Sweden. In many cases, diet and lifestyle are implicated. Differences in smoking rates, for example, would explain any variations in lung cancer rates, while the arrival of refrigeration, and the resulting decline in salted, smoked and pickled foods, is linked to the drop in stomach cancer rates. Western diets, high in energy and saturated and other unhealthy fats, but low in essential fatty acids and protective antioxidants, are also blamed for the risk in cancer and other diseases.

But in some cases there are variations in cancer rates between areas that have pretty much the same diets and lifestyles, and which cannot be explained by known factors. One such mystery is why the Arctic regions – Greenland, Alaska and northern Canada – have very low levels of some hormone-dependent cancers, especially breast, but also ovarian and prostate cancer.

Researchers from the University of Cologne say it has been argued that the low breast cancer risk in the Arctic regions is a result of not having a Western lifestyle. But, they say, recently increased risks for tobacco, alcohol and diet-related cancers in those countries suggest Western lifestyles have already arrived. In any case, they point out, the idea that high-fat diets explain higher rates of breast cancer is questionable because dietary fat content has been pretty much the same as those in the West since around 1930.

So, if diet and lifestyle cannot explain the difference, what can?

One of the big differences between the Arctic areas and elsewhere, of course, is natural light. Those living north of the Arctic Circle experience large seasonal variations in light. Every year, there are periods when the sun does not rise above the horizon for several weeks, and there are seasonal periods of continuous darkness or daylight.

The hormone melatonin, secreted in the pineal gland, responds to light and dark, and has also been implicated in breast cancer. Melatonin is produced in larger quantities when there is no light, and research has suggested that exposure to modern lighting at night means low levels. A number of studies indicate that low melatonin levels are associated with increases in certain types of hormone-dependent cancers, including breast and prostate cancer.

The Cologne team suggests that in the Arctic Circle reduced exposure to light boosts pineal gland production and reduces the risk of hormone-dependent cancers. The argument is that over the year as a whole, there is a net increase in melatonin. "We predict that, if the hypothesis is valid, the excess protective melatonin among people living north of the Arctic Circle reduces their risk of hormone-dependent cancers, as compared with people living south of this boundary," they say.

6

HAIRSPRAY, HAIRINESS AND OTHER CAUSES OF CANCER

Lights at night cause cancer

TURN OFF THE LIGHT, UNPLUG the TV, draw the curtains and get out the sleeping masks … and you might just live longer.

Turning off the lights may not just be good for global warming, saving the planet and reducing your carbon footprint, it may also lower the risk of cancer. In modern times, most people spend almost all their waking day and night bathed in natural or artificial lights of one kind or another, vastly different from the kind of environment in which the human body and body clock evolved. Back in those days, it was all very different. Things were pretty much black and white, with light during the day and blackness at night. That meant life was straightforward for the body clock and its main enforcer, the hormone melatonin, which is produced by the pineal gland in response to darkness and which helps us to know when to sleep and when to wake up.

Production of the hormone peaks in the middle of the night, then slowly falls away in the run-up to dawn. Production of the hormone is inhibited by light, and that means excessive light at night may result in the body not getting enough of the hormone, which also has an important role as a disease-fighting antioxidant. Some animal studies have suggested that melatonin may prevent damage to DNA caused by the development of some cancers.

Stephen Pauley, a researcher from Idaho, says that the suppression of melatonin by exposure to light at night may be one reason for the higher rates of breast and colorectal cancers in the developed world and that the theory deserves more attention. He says evidence now exists that links exposure to light at night to breast and colon cancers in shift workers. He points out that modern lights emit more blue wavelengths than the early gas, kerosene and incandescent lamps, and that blue light is thought to be more effective in blocking melatonin.

Pauley says precautionary action needs to start now and all lighting fixtures should be designed to minimize interference with the normal circadian rhythm. We should sleep in total darkness, use non-glare, non-blue outdoor and indoor lights, and offices should have natural daylight, or, if that's not possible, full-spectrum white light.

Indoor night lighting should be dim, and wavelengths should be shifted towards the yellow and orange. Read by incandescent lights rather than fluorescents, and TVs should not be left on when we're asleep. Blinds should be closed if there is street lighting, and shift workers should sleep during the day in total darkness with the help of a sleep mask.

"Until more research directly links exposure to light at night to increased rates of human cancers, it may be wise to consider preventive measures in the application of everyday lighting practices," says the researcher. "Shift workers should be advised that preliminary studies now indicate that there are health risks associated with work performed in the early morning hours, and that the risk of breast and colorectal cancer increases as the number of days of shift work increase."

Dogs give women breast cancer

MUCH REMAINS TO BE DISCOVERED about the origins of breast cancer, but could it really be true that keeping a dog increases the risk of the disease?

According to research at the University of Munich, dogs may pick up a virus from mice and pass it on to humans. They found that 8 out of 10 women diagnosed with cancer had close contacts with dogs at some time. "Published results and our own observations lead us to propose that dogs may harbour carcinogenic risk factors," they say.

Breast cancer is an increasing problem. Environmental factors of various kinds have been blamed for the majority of cases, with only 5–10 per cent considered to be hereditary. A number of viruses have already been implicated, including Epstein-Barr and the human papilloma virus, which is also involved in cervical cancer.

Analysis of breast cancer cases by the Munich researchers showed that patients with cancer of the breast were significantly more likely to have kept a dog than a cat. In fact, 79.7 per cent of all patients had intensive contact with dogs before they were diagnosed. Only 4.4 per cent of the patients did not have pets at any time compared to 57.3 per cent of a healthy control group. This, say the researchers, shows a 29-fold increased risk for pet owners.

The researchers also point to a study in Norway which reported a very high level – 53.3 per cent – of breast cancers in 14,401 dogs. The team then looked at what virus could be common to both dogs and humans. The one they homed in on is the mouse mammary tumour virus (MMTV) which triggers breast cancer in mice and which has been investigated for possible links to human breast cancer. The theory is that dogs, and possibly other pets, harbour and transmit MMTV or MMTV-like viruses that can induce human breast cancer.

One of the suggestions is that the dog, an animal that has frequent close contacts with humans, picks up the virus from a mouse and then passes it on to humans. Dogs, say the researchers, follow the trail of animals with their nose on the ground and could inhale infectious excretions, including those from mice.

The researchers say that the theory may help to explain why women from Eastern countries are at increased risk of breast cancer when they move to Western nations: "Asian or Oriental women seldom keep dogs as pets. Migration to Western countries may change their lifestyle, including keeping pet dogs. This might contribute to the increased incidence of breast cancer in these women after their move to the West." They add, "Transmission of MMTV or a MMTV-like virus or bacterial risk factors by pet dogs offers a possible explanation for the increased incidence of breast cancer in Western countries and its correlation with a higher living standard."

It's suggested that development of a tumour vaccine against dog breast cancer could help in the search for a human breast cancer vaccine.

Electric typewriters cause breast cancer

SAMUEL MILHAM WAS MEASURING MAGNETIC fields when he stumbled across a curious finding. Readings taken around many of the electric typewriters in the offices where he was working were generating a very high magnetic field. While most other places in the offices measured 2 mG or less, readings around some typewriters soared to 100 mG.

At the time he thought little of it, but some years later when he was looking at an analysis of the jobs of more than 9,000 women diagnosed with breast cancer, he found the possibility of a link with his magnetic field research. In the job group that included secretaries and typists there were far more deaths than were statistically expected. Taking into account age and general risk factors, there should have been 592 deaths. There were in fact 774. Further analysis showed that most female occupations associated with typing had increased breast cancer mortality.

Intrigued, he and colleagues in the Washington State Health Department carried out further tests in typewriter repair shops in four western US cities. What they found was that a number of the machines had magnetic fields up to 400 mG. At breast level, the working height for typists, the fields ranged up to 50 mG. Nine of 16 measured machines had magnetic fields above 5 mG at user breast level and 5 of 16 machines had magnetic fields above 40 mG at that level.

The researchers, who say that power frequency magnetic fields have been associated with both male and female breast cancer, point out that typewriters have now been largely replaced by computers which generate much lower magnetic fields. "However, with the long latency times of human solid tumours, it is possible that some newly diagnosed breast cancer cases could be due to past exposure to magnetic fields from electric typewriters. In future studies of breast cancer, a question dealing with electric typewriter use should be included," they say.

Hairy people have less cancer

STOP SHAVING, WAXING AND TRIMMING those hairs and you might be less likely to get cancer.

The modern trend of removing facial, head and body hair could be hazardous to health because it may be there to protect lymph nodes under the skin from ultraviolet radiation from the sun, according to this research.

Research by Dr Svetlana Komarova, from McGill University, Canada suggests that there are striking similarities between the pattern of facial hair and the distribution of superficial lymph nodes. That suggests a potential role for facial hair as a protector of lymph nodes and the thyroid, and that's important, she says, because of the established link between nodes and cancers.

"The position of contemporary fashion towards body hair includes social pressure for removal of axillary and bikini line hair for women, facial hair for men and even body hair for men. If this hypothesis is proven to be true, the implications will be significant," she says.

While it is accepted that hair or fur on animals has a protective effect, there is no such consensus about human hair. In fact, says Komarova, dermatologists maintain that hair has no vital function in humans. But what if hair does have a protective purpose? To answer this question, Komarova first looked at what it could be covering up, and the answer she came up with was the lymph nodes, the glands which play a key role in orchestrating the immune system against disease and infection. They produce lymph, a fluid which travels throughout the body filtering impurities, and are found in the groin, armpits, neck, under the jaw and chin, and on the back of the head. All of these areas, as Komarova points out, are covered by hair.

It is also known that lymph nodes are involved in cancer. When cancerous cells break away from a tumour, they can travel in the lymphatic system to another part of the body where they may grow as secondary tumours.

Having found something that hair could be protecting, Komarova then looked at what it could be protecting the nodes from. She analysed a number of candidates, including the cold, but opted for heat and ultraviolet radiation from direct sunlight, a known cause of cancer.

But if hair is so important, why don't women have facial hair, and why do men become bald?

It's suggested that the lack of facial hair in women may be because the female hormone oestrogen lowers the risk of sun damage in women and so they do not need so much hair, or because the male hormone testosterone increases vulnerability, which is why men need that extra hairy barrier between them and the sun.

The second potential weakness of the theory – baldness – is also dealt with. The nodes on the head, it's suggested, have another protective barrier, the skull, which makes the evolutionary necessity for head hair less important. Secondly, it's argued, a little bit of radiation could be good for the brain. It may be no coincidence that bald men have been shown to be more intelligent. The link between the sun, brain and intelligence could make baldness a desirable evolutionary trait in some circumstances.

"Thus, I propose the hypothesis that human hair serves a vital function of protecting the brain, genitalia and lymph nodes from damage by the sun and heat exposure," says Komarova. "This hypothesis calls for studies aimed at the role of facial hair in males, strongly suggesting that fair-skinned men would benefit from having facial hair. If confirmed, this hypothesis will have a major impact not only in medicine, but also in social fashion, economics, and arts."

Quitting smoking too fast triggers lung cancer

A CURIOUS FINDING EMERGED when doctors reviewed all the cases of lung cancer that they had worked on. Each of the patients had a history of smoking of course, but what was unusual was that most of them had quit the habit in the months just before they were diagnosed.

Struck by the relationship between the timing of the appearance of the cancer and an abrupt and recent cessation of smoking in many cases, the doctors delved more deeply into the backgrounds of the patients. What they found was that over a period of four years a total of 312 cases had been treated for lung cancer, and of those, 182 patients had stopped smoking 5–15 months before being diagnosed.

Each of the patients, aged between 47 and 74 years, had been addicted to the habit for at least 25 years, smoking in excess of 20 cigarettes a day. In order to give up, the men and women had to have smoked, and there is no doubt that smoking causes cancer. According to Cancerbackup, Europe's leading cancer information charity, it is the cause of most lung cancers, and although lung cancer can also develop in people who do not smoke, it is much rarer, and the risk of developing lung cancer increases with the number of cigarettes smoked. Filtered and low tar cigarettes may slightly reduce the risk of developing cancer, although it is still far greater than that of a non-smoker.

But is it possible that suddenly giving up somehow triggers or speeds up the growth of cancer? Can it be that such a sudden physical change after a quarter of century of smoking catches the body's defence systems off guard?

Researchers in Mangalore, India say the abrupt ending of the habit may lead to the body repair system going out of control, triggering uncontrolled cell division and the growth of tumours. One theory is that when smoking is stopped, there is a surge in body repair activity on the lining of the cells damaged by years of tobacco use, but that the level of repair work is so great it gets out of control.

The researchers say this raises questions about whether addicts should be weaned or tapered off tobacco instead of being advised to giving up smoking overnight. Perhaps, they suggest, the immune and repair systems should be given time to adjust to the withdrawal.

"The striking direct statistical correlation between cessation of smoking to the development of lung malignancies, more than 60 per cent, is too glaring to be dismissed as coincidental," they say. "It is our premise that a surge and spurt in re-activation of bodily healing and repair mechanisms of chronic smoke-damaged respiratory tissue is induced and spurred by an abrupt discontinuation of habit, goes awry, triggering uncontrolled cell division and tumour."

They say that larger studies and more extensive reviews of case histories of lung cancer patients are needed to throw more light on the issue. They add, "No doubt, tobacco kills too many. Or does it?"

Cancer is best diagnosed in the summer

PEOPLE DIAGNOSED WITH SOME CANCERS are less likely to survive if they are diagnosed in the winter.

According to research at the Institute for Cancer Research, Oslo, the risk of dying during the following 18 months is 30–50 per cent lower for cases diagnosed during summer and autumn compared with winter. Similar effects have been found for a number of cancers, including breast, lung, colon, Hodgkin's lymphoma and prostate. All showed the same trend, with a winter diagnosis leading to a higher risk of death.

Just what could be at work is not clear, but the seasonal differences suggested that sun, or heat or cold, or some other factor that changes with the seasons, may be at work.

The first suspect was vitamin D. We get most of this vitamin from the sun, and ultraviolet radiation in particular; but it is not around at the levels we need during the winter. Vitamin D is known to promote good bone health and has been associated with other health benefits, but could it really have such a substantial impact on the development of a major disease like cancer?

In the search for other candidates, the Norwegian team investigated folate or folic acid, the B vitamin which women are advised to take during pregnancy to avoid neural tube defects in their child. Folate is necessary for the production of new cells and is especially important for the growing foetus. Intriguingly, the rate of children born with such defects, which are closely related to folate deficiency, also varies with the season.

The rationale behind the season-of-diagnosis theory is that solar radiation can degrade folate so that cell division is slowed. This, it's suggested, hits cancer cells hardest, because they expand the fastest.

Animal experiments support the idea, showing that folate deficiency does indeed delay tumour progression and that ultraviolet light degrades folate. Seasonal variations of folate have also been seen in psoriasis patients undergoing ultraviolet-based light therapy.

The researchers say their work shows that folate and its synthetic form, folic acid, are sensitive to ultraviolet radiation. They point out that the evolutionary reason for the brown skin colour of people living near the equator is protection of folate in the blood from sun-induced degradation.

"The observed seasonal variation in the survival rate of several types of cancer in Norway is due to photodegradation of folate by sun exposure. The folate levels in the serum of these patients may be lower in summer and autumn than in winter," they say. "If our hypothesis is correct, sun-induced degradation of blood folate might act beneficially with regard to cancer prognosis. Studies examining blood levels of folate at the moment of diagnosis in relation to subsequent death risk appear warranted."

Hairsprays cause cancer

ONE OF THE MANY MYSTERIES about breast cancer is why there are such wide differences between the numbers of cases and deaths among different ethnic groups in the same country.

Many of the known risk factors for the disease – age at menarche, menopause and first baby, and number of relatives with breast cancer, as well as gene mutations, obesity and excessive alcohol consumption – are common to all groups. Yet African-American women have very different risk rates from white women. Overall, they are less likely to develop breast cancer than white women, but at any age they are more likely to die from it. And the incidence of the disease in African-American women aged 20–29 years is nearly 50 per cent higher than for white women of the same age. African-American women under the age of 40 also have a higher incidence of breast cancer than do whites, although they tend to have more children earlier in life, which in white women is a factor that actually lowers the risk of cancer.

With the exception of inherited genes that increase the risk of disease, most of the known risk factors for breast cancer are related to a build-up of exposure to oestrogens, and a woman's lifetime risk of breast cancer increases with greater exposure to oestrogens. So could there be any differences in exposure that might explain the difference in prevalence of breast cancer between races? Are African-American women exposed to more oestrogens, and, if so, what could be responsible?

According to researchers at the University of Pittsburgh Cancer Institute, New York University and University of Texas, widely used personal care products – hair sprays and skin products that contain hormones or placenta – may well be the culprit.

African-American women could be at greater risk, it's suggested, because they use more of these products. The researchers say there is evidence that African-American adults and children use personal care products containing hormones 6–10 times more frequently than whites do. For treatment of hair and skin, African-American females may start using them earlier, as infants and toddlers, and they also may be exposed in the womb when their mothers use the products during pregnancy.

The theory is that the oestrogen in the products gets into breast tissue either in early life or while the baby is still in the womb. Once in the tissue, it may stimulate breast bud development in early life, increasing the risk of disease later.

The researchers say that several reports have shown that oestrogen-containing products can result in premature sexual development in infants or toddlers. In one case, an ointment containing oestrogens on diapers caused early sexual development in an eight-month-old child.

"These *in utero*, early life and ongoing lifetime exposures to oestrogens and xenoestrogens and xenohormones could account in part for the higher incidence of breast cancer in young African-American women. Continued exposure may also contribute to the increased lethality of breast cancer in both younger and older African-American women," say the researchers. They add, "People have a right to know whether products they use on themselves or their children contain compounds that may increase their risk of disease, including cancer. Under current policy in many countries that right is denied.

"As a matter of public health policy, manufacturers should be required to provide information on current and past inclusion of hormones in their PCPs [personal care products]. In the meantime, parents and guardians should be advised to avoid using any products on children that are known or suspected to contain hormones and/or placenta."

Skin colour and breast cancer

IT HAS BEEN KNOWN for some time that oestrogen plays a key role in the development of breast cancer.

Women who menstruate early, before the age of 12, and those going into menopause late, after 55, or who have their first child after age 35, or who have no children at all, are at a higher risk of developing the disease. The link in each of these is believed to be oestrogen and many breast cancer drugs work by blocking the female hormone. Oestrogen receptors are found on up to 80 per cent of breast tumours, and around 60 per cent respond to hormone-based treatments. But it's also thought that foetuses exposed to higher levels of oestrogen may be at a higher lifetime risk of breast cancer too.

While age at menarche and menopause, and number of children, are easy to establish and the risk calculated, the problem with foetal exposure is that there is no apparent way of knowing what it was … but then again, perhaps there is.

According to researchers from the University of Central Lancashire, skin colour may be the answer. The theory is that relative skin colour within each racial group may be a marker of foetal exposure. The lighter the skin, relative to people of the same overall skin colour, the greater oestrogen exposure and therefore the higher the breast cancer risk.

While pigmentation of the face and exposed parts of the body increases in response to UV light, so-called constitutive pigmentation, which is measured from the inner surface of the upper arm, is strongly influenced by genes.

"We suggest that constitutive skin colour in women is a marker for prenatal and adult oestrogen levels such that within ethnic groups light-skinned women have experienced higher *in utero* and adult oestrogen than dark-skinned women," they say. "Scores for constitutive skin pigment may therefore be predictive of risk for breast cancer and low scores could be used to identify individuals at high risk."

The researchers say there are sex differences in skin colour that suggest pigmentation is influenced by oestrogen and testosterone, and that in all societies women tend to be lighter-skinned than men. The gender difference becomes more obvious at puberty when women's skin becomes lighter and men's darker. Women's skin may be lighter because they have more fat under the skin which is a source of oestrogen.

Support for the theory comes from another marker of hormone exposure in the womb, the ratio of the lengths of the second (index) finger and the fourth (ring) finger. A relatively long ring finger is a sign that the foetus was exposed to higher levels of testosterone, while a relatively long index finger is a marker of increased oestrogen exposure

Research shows that women with a lighter skin are also likely to have a longer index finger. Intriguingly, and to complete the circle, vulnerability to early breast cancer has also been associated with a relatively long index finger.

The researchers say that in future research, colour scores should be taken from patients with breast cancer and from age-matched healthy controls and compared: "It is predicted that the former will be lighter than the latter. Light skin may also be predictive of early age of presentation of the tumour, the presence of oestrogen receptors on the tumour and rapid progression of the disease." It could also be helpful in the treatment of the disease, because women with lighter skins may be more likely to respond to oestrogen-blocking drugs.

7

HOW TO CURE
MOST THINGS
AND GET TALLER

A cure for constipation

CONSTIPATION IS A SIGNIFICANT, and unpleasant, health problem with as many as one in three of us suffering at some time.

It's defined as a difficulty in passing stools, and it may include pain during bowel movements, an inability to empty bowels after straining or pushing for more than 10 minutes, or no bowel movements at all for more than three days. Common causes include a low-fibre diet, lack of physical activity and not drinking enough water. Stress, depression, pregnancy, diet changes and travel can make symptoms worse.

Over the years a huge range of treatments have been suggested, ranging from liquorice, figs and boiled green cabbage leaves, to radishes, bran and cocoa. There are also many over-the-counter laxatives, as well as psychological therapy and biofeedback. Some of them work for some people some of the time, but new treatments are sorely needed for a condition that affects more than two million people in the UK at any one time.

It had been thought that there was little else to try, but researchers at Tehran University of Medical Sciences, Iran have come up with an idea which could solve the problem, at least for half the population.

Their theory is that rubbing the top of the penis, the glans, while trying to defecate might just do the trick. The idea is that squeezing the glans leads to the contraction of key muscles in the general genital and anal areas. In particular, it sets up a reflex action known as the bulbocavernosus reflex around the anal area. That, it's suggested, results in a contraction of anal muscles and a build-up of inner pressures, thus triggering the urge to get the bowel moving.

"It seems that squeezing the glans during defecation could result in contraction of anal sphincter, increasing rectal pressure which subsequently stimulates rectal sensory nerves that produce an urge to defecate," say the researchers. "So this easy manoeuvre could improve the defecation process and reduce constipation incidence. Surely, the efficacy of this manoeuvre should be assessed in clinical trials."

Nuts cure toothache

IT'S NOT JUST IN SCIENCE FICTION novels and horror movies that scientists experiment on themselves. Over the years, many scientific breakthroughs have been made because researchers have been prepared to experiment on themselves in an attempt to discover causes and treatments for a wide range of conditions, including cholera and yellow fever.

The dentist Horace Wells tested the effects of nitrous oxide by having one or two of his teeth extracted while breathing in the gas; William Morton, a pioneer of anaesthesia, almost died during his experimentation; Jesse Lazear inoculated himself with tropical diseases; and Werner Forssman tested catheters by inserting one into his arm and pushing it towards his heart.

In more recent times, Barry Marshall deliberately infected himself with a newly discovered strain of bacteria, *Helicobacter pylori*. He was sick for days, but the results of his experiment changed the way stomach ulcers are treated. For that work, Marshall and colleague, Robin Warren, won the Nobel Prize for Medicine.

Headlines may have been made by pioneering scientists like these, but many others, working in less glamorous and less dangerous areas, have also been prepared to put themselves on the line.

In that same honourable tradition of self-experimentation, Charles Weber from North Carolina put his oral health on the line when he tried cashew nuts as a cure for an abscess under a tooth. He says research shows that Gram-positive bacteria, which cause tooth decay, acne, tuberculosis and leprosy, are killed by chemicals in cashew apples, cashew shell oil and probably cashew nuts.

The suggestion is that the active chemicals in the nuts are anacardic acids, which in test tube experiments appear to be active against *Streptococcus mutans*, the cause of tooth decay. According to Weber, the acid can be lethal to bacteria in 15 minutes: "I have made raw cashew nuts the main part of my diet for 24 h on four occasions and have eliminated an abscessed tooth each time. There were no obvious side-effects. A fifth time required several days. It is possible that just eating a couple of ounces each day for a week or so would work also and might avoid any intolerance or allergy to cashew nuts," he says.

Leather shoes cure diseases

IT WAS AN UNUSUAL EXPERIMENT, but would it work? Could standing in leather-soled shoes sprinkled with magnesium sulphate set up an electric current flowing up one leg and down the other that would improve bone health and tackle gout and arthritis?

In a four-month, one-man trial, the 57-year old volunteer put magnesium in his shoes to see what happened. Not only was there a general improvement in his health, including better breathing, he lost 20 pounds in weight.

According to the theory of this Tasmania-based researcher, it's all to do with electrolytic activity and the flow of electric currents through the body. The theory is that this flow has an effect on the chemical balance of the body, including boosting energy.

The concept is that when this natural current is allowed to flow it brings about far-reaching effects in health, including improvement in bone, as well as helping to control uric acid-linked diseases like gout. According to the theory, the electron flow travels up one leg and down the other when both bare feet are on the ground, with the feet acting as electrodes.

Initial tests with steel pegs in the ground showed that there was indeed a small current flow. But two questions remained – would the electrical resistance of the human body be too great to allow current to flow from one foot to the other foot via the legs, and would the foot act in the same way as a steel peg?

To answer these questions, the investigator placed two stainless steel plates on the ground. When the experimenter stood on them wearing plastic-soled shoes there was no current flow, but when his feet were bare, current did indeed flow up one leg and down the other. The third trial, involving wearing leather shoes, showed that leather, a better conductor of electricity than plastic, also allowed a current to flow.

But could it have an effect on disease? To find out, experiments were carried out to see whether uric acid, which is known to be involved in a number of diseases, could be broken down by passing the same small level of electricity through it.

In one test, a constant current was passed through a solution of uric acid using stainless steel plates as electrodes. After 24 hours a brown deposit began to form in the bottom of the beaker, suggesting a chemical change was occurring. It is possible, says the researcher, that the same process could be happening in the body to control diseases that stem from the build-up of uric acid. Unfortunately, changes in the manufacture of footwear over the years has led to more plastic-soled shoes being worn, which means people may not be getting as much benefit as they would from wearing leather. The answer, say the report, is to buy leather-soled shoes, or wear shoes with chemically treated inner soles that conduct electricity.

"The cost of a changeover to shoes with conducting soles to allow current to flow with its benefits to general health would only be small," says the report. "It is now reasonable to conclude that it is possible under natural conditions for a current flow to take place in the body due to the bare feet being in contact with the ground. It is suggested that if this natural current is allowed to flow it would bring about far-reaching effects in health generally, improvement in bone structure, and help in controlling uric acid diseases, arthritis and nervous disorders."

A cure for hiccups

ALMOST EVERYONE GETS HICCUPS at some time. For most people it lasts a few seconds or minutes, but for others it can go on for hours, days, and even weeks.

Hiccups are caused by involuntary contractions of the diaphragm, the muscle that separates the chest from the abdomen, and the classic hic sound is the result of the sudden sealing of the trachea by the closure of the epiglottis. It's purpose is unknown, but because it's universal – it's even been observed in foetuses – there ought to be an evolutionary explanation for it, and many theories have been advanced. It has been suggested that it could be a relic of a distant aquatic past where it stopped water getting into the lungs, or that it could be a remnant of a primitive sucking reflex.

Whatever the cause, it can be an unpleasant, embarrassing and in some cases long and painful experience, and the search for a cure has been going on for centuries. During that time many diverse, even bizarre treatments have been suggested, including gargling with water, a slap on the back, a tot of whisky, blowing a balloon, a teaspoon of sugar, a cold spoon on the back and, more recently, a spoonful of peanut butter and an ice cream.

Although some work for some people, none has proved to be a panacea. But researchers at Kasturba Medical College, India may at last have found one – putting a finger into the throat of the hiccupping victim.

"A simple technique I have tried with success on many is initiating the gag reflex. Just reach out digitally to the base of the tongue and depress it slightly, and even intractable hiccups disappears," according to the report. "Whatever the root or rationale of the digital intervention, as a simple and easily performable first aid method, use of the gag reflex may save the unfortunate intractable hiccup sufferer from unease and tension."

Just how it works is not clear, but the gag reflex is a contraction of the back of the throat designed to prevent choking. Touching the soft palate or base of the tongue, or even attempting to, triggers a strong reflex action in most people. One theory is that the shock or sudden change in breathing that occurs as a result of the reflex action somehow re-sets the nerves that are involved in hiccups. Another is that because the mind is focused on the reflex action it forgets about the hiccups and thereby breaks the cycle.

Humming 120 times a day cures blocked noses

CHRONIC RHINOSINUSITIS IS A MAJOR health problem affecting an estimated 50 million Americans and Europeans. A chronic inflammatory disease of the nasal passages and the sinuses that can last for longer than three months, its symptoms include a blocked nose, breathing difficulties and a reduced sense of smell, as well as the formation of nasal polyps in more severe cases.

Just what causes it is not clear, although a study at the Mayo Clinic, Minnesota points to a fungus inside the nose as the culprit. In its efforts to zap the fungus, the immune system seems to trigger an inflammatory response that results in a runny nose, cough, sore throat, pain in the teeth and headache.

Treatments that have been used to tackle the symptoms include antibiotics, painkillers, corticosteroids and surgery to clear blocked nasal passages, but a cure has yet to be found.

If fungus is responsible, one of the ways to treat it could be to use nitric oxide. Toxic to bacteria and fungi, the gas is naturally released in the human respiratory tract, so in theory it should be the way to kill the fungus. But how do you get high enough concentrations at the site of the fungal infection?

The answer is simple: hum. According to researcher George Eby of Texas, levels of nasal nitric oxide are increased 15- to 20-fold by humming. In his research he cites the first case report of a man cured by humming. The 64-year-old had rhinosinusitis with severe headache, cough and insomnia, and he had tried everything – steroid shots, aspirin, zinc lozenges, antihistamines, decongestants and antibiotics – but they either didn't work at all or were minimally effective.

It was then that he tried humming. Not just any humming, it had to be at the right frequency and done at regular intervals. Low frequency humming, around 130 Hz, apparently produces the greatest amount of nitric oxide.

He hummed strongly for one hour at a rate of 18 hums a minute at bedtime the first night, and hummed strongly at a low pitch between 60 and 120 times in four sessions a day for the following four days. The humming was seen to increase nasal vibrations.

The morning after the first humming session, the man awoke with a clear nose and was breathing easily. The only side-effect with the treatment was dizziness that can be brought on by excessively vigorous humming.

According to the report, half an hour of humming might also help with symptoms of the common cold. "By humming 60–120 times, four times per day – including a session at bedtime

— symptoms were essentially eliminated in four days. There is now hope that the humming method will be highly effective in treating patients with little or no other medical or surgical treatment required after diagnosis," says the report. It warns, however, that small women and children may need to take care: "The ability to strongly vibrate the nose by humming may be diminished by small facial features, suggesting that small women and children may need to work harder than men in managing the condition with humming."

Drivers too need to exercise caution: "The side effect of excessively strong and frequent humming — dizziness — precludes humming from being used while driving a motor vehicle or doing activities that require full concentration."

Magnets can make you taller

MUCH MONEY IS SPENT ANNUALLY on pills and potions and exercise programmes designed to make short people taller. There are supplements that claim to add inches to height, stretching exercises that make similar claims, and diverse techniques which are said to work by triggering the release of natural hormones involved in growth. Sadly, in many cases the only thing they stretch is the imagination. The one certain way to get taller is to have a painful operation during which the legs bones are broken and pulled apart, causing new bone to grow and bridge the gap. It involves traumatic orthopaedic surgery, is painful, expensive and takes a long time, and is reserved for the very short.

But in societies where height is esteemed, and where shortness is seen as a substantial disadvantage in mating potential, employment prospects and a number of other areas, demand for a quick-fix, grow-tall remedy has always been high. To cater for that demand, doctors in India have come up with what they believe is a novel, painless and relatively cheap way of getting taller. All it involves is magnets strapped to the legs.

The theory is quite simple. While magnets can be used to attract, in this application they are used to repel. The treatment involves strapping two powerful ring magnets onto the outside of the leg or thigh that needs to be lengthened, leaving a small gap between them. The magnets are strapped in place so that their repelling poles are facing each other, either side of the gap. The effect is such that if they were not firmly strapped on the legs, the magnets would be physically pushed apart. The theory is that because they cannot move, the gap – and the leg bone – has to grow. In other words, the repulsive fields trigger the bone into increasing its length.

The researchers at Kasturba Medical College says they have started experimental studies that show it may work: "The exact magnetic pressure, the length of treatment, the bone selected (femur or tibia), all are alterable to suit the patient's convenience and pleasure. We have no doubt that, with further experimentation, we should be able to improve and standardize the specific requirements of the procedure to enable the best possible results," they say.

They suggest that magnets could have other applications in bone growth and even in the repair of fractures, and research at the University of California supports that claim. Researchers there have used a remarkable new magnetic treatment for correcting sunken chests in children. The magnets, one implanted in the breast bone, the other in a garment worn over the chest for up to three months, are attracted to each other and as a result the chest is slowly pulled out. Doctors who are pioneering the therapy say it could revolutionize treatment for the condition and replace conventional surgery which involves several days in hospital and weeks or months convalescing.

Drinking water lowers the risk of heart disease

THOSE MUCH MALIGNED FATTY DEPOSITS on the walls of arteries may be innocent after all.

In fact, the deposits blamed for hardening of the arteries or atherosclerosis, and the resulting higher risk of heart disease and stroke, may simply be trying to defend the body.

It seems it's not so much the fat we eat as the temperature of the chest that's to blame for the furring up of blood vessels. Eating calorie-dense food, it's suggested, raises the temperature of the chest and abdomen and when the heat does not go away, the abdominal and coronary arteries use lipid or fat as an insulator to line the arteries to try to keep the body temperature from rising.

However, that unwanted temperature rise could be prevented by drinking water: "The water should be drunk during, or just before or after the meal to reduce the osmolality of the food. It is imperative that the water consumption should be higher in warmer conditions," says the researcher from the State of California Department of Health Services.

Atherosclerosis occurs when deposits of fatty substances, including cholesterol, build up a fatty layer on the inside of an artery. That can reduce blood flow and also lead to the formation of blood clots that can trigger a heart attack or a stroke. It is a leading cause of mortality worldwide, and some research suggests it is triggered by initial damage to the artery tissue, with high levels of cholesterol, diabetes, smoking and high blood pressure taking the blame.

The California researcher says that although several theories have been suggested, none can fully explain the development of the disease, and that it is time for a paradigm shift in thinking. According to the report, there is ample scientific evidence that calorie-dense food does raise temperatures. Research on animals, for instance, shows that eating fructose raises temperatures in the colon, while drinking water does not. The report says that if this heat is not removed, it will raise body as well as blood temperature. It says it is difficult for the body then to get rid of heat around the chest and abdomen because of high levels of fat in those areas.

According to the theory, the aorta, the largest artery in the body, insulates itself from the heat by depositing fatty material on the walls. And it is that that leads to atherosclerosis, not eating fat: "Fat ingestion does not cause excessive thermogenesis, and therefore does not cause atherosclerosis. Both skinny as well as obese people are at risk of developing atherosclerosis," says the report.

If heat is the cause, then water could be a new therapy for avoiding heart disease. Not only does it cool the abdomen and chest, it also absorbs the excess heat produced and removes it from the body in urine. The report recommends that 1–1.5 ml of water should be consumed per kcal of energy expenditure. "This is a new and convincing hypothesis which is backed by scientific research," it adds.

A cure for most diseases

ALTHOUGH ALMOST EVERYONE HAS BEEN on a diet or plans to go on one at some time, global rates of obesity and diseases associated with overweight are at record levels. In some countries obesity rates are now nudging 20 per cent or more, and the proportion of the population who are either obese or overweight is in excess of half, making thinness a minority trait.

Some evidence suggests that dieting doesn't really work, or that it works for some people for a little of the time, but that it is not really effective overall. And that's a problem because it means the diseases that are linked to being overweight, ranging from cancer, heart disease and diabetes to hypertension, snoring and infertility, are likely to continue to rise.

What's needed is a highly effective diet, one that tackles the root cause of why we are getting fat, helps us lose weight and prevents or even cures diseases. But what could it be?

Step forward the chimp diet.

In a research letter, "Healthiest diet hypothesis: how to cure most diseases", Hans Dehmelt of the University of Washington suggests that a return to eating raw food may be the answer. He says that from the earliest times to about five million years ago, man's ancient primate ancestors lived exclusively in the deep tropical forests of southern Africa on a diet that carefully evolved over a period of about 20 million years. But then, adventurous members ventured out into the surrounding savannah and started to eat meat by scavenging the carcasses of large grazing animals brought down by predators. These meat-eaters, he suggests, were probably the start of the lineage that led to *Homo sapiens*.

"As we multiplied, this pattern repeated, and again and again we were forced to subsist on even less and less desirable diets until today a large fraction of the population has adopted variations of the Big Mac diet," he says. But those who stayed in the forests and on the local diet changed very little and became *Homo troglodytes*, the chimpanzee, and man's closest relative. The raw diet of the chimps is 75 per cent ripe wild fruit, 20 per cent leaves and pith, and five per cent foods of animal origin. Essential fatty acids, now known to protect against a wide range of diseases in man, including cancer and heart disease, contribute nearly half of the fat in the chimp diet.

Dehmelt says that this remains the healthiest diet for man because 20 million years of evolution mean that he is still best adapted to it. "Common ancestors of Man and Chimp did not cook their foods. All later diets up to the current Big Mac diet of the broad American masses increasingly rely on foodstuffs such as meat, grains, beans and potatoes that have to be made edible by cooking," says the report. "Consequently, all are less healthy. Approximating the chimp diet by suitably supplemented super-market items may give us the best of both worlds."

A cure for death

PORTRAITS IN THE ATTIC, fountains of youth, Never-Never Land, Peter Pan, elixirs of eternal life … man has always been obsessed with the pursuit of youth, longevity and the Holy Grail – living forever. Or as Woody Allen put it, "Some people want to achieve immor-tality through their works or their descendants. I prefer to achieve immortality by not dying."

Medicine is rooted in the idea of delaying death, while reli-gions have prospered on offering life after death. The ancient Egyptians tried to fight death with mummification, and some modern millionaires have plans for their bodies to be frozen after death in the hope of waking up again in a few hundred years when a cure for their terminal illness has been discovered.

But is death really inevitable?

"A simple philosophical consideration of the nature of our lives as individual human beings suggests an astounding possibil-ity – that death may be preventable using technology which has existed for centuries," says researcher Charles Olson of Delaware.

His theory is that the body-freezers or cryo-preservers are on the right track, but have missed the point. Death can be cheated not be defrosting old brains, but by using chemically preserved organs as a blueprint for making an exact copy.

The mind is, he says, fundamental to life. The brain is the computer and the mind, the act of computing. The unique, indi-vidual design of the brain is crucial to the working of the mind and has to be preserved if there is any hope of eternal life. His theory is that if the brain is the machine and the mind the information-processing software, why can't the latter be transferred to another machine just as software travels between computers? After all, he says, brain tissue is constantly renewing itself, and most of the molecules we die with were not there when we were born. The substitution of new brain machine for old is, he suggests, simply a more sudden and complete version of the turnover that occurs naturally.

By preserving the brain chemically after death, the blueprint for the mind will be preserved forever – neither dead nor alive, just waiting. Then, in the future, perhaps 100 centuries from now, the blueprint will be read and a new machine, a new brain, will be created to house the mind.

"A preserved brain may in fact be an individual in a state of suspended animation, not in a biological sense but rather in the sense related to consciousness and the mind. Just as anaesthesia temporarily halts our lives as conscious individuals, so brain preservation allows a lengthy but ultimately temporary halt in conscious life, like a long, deep and dreamless sleep," says the report. "From the narrow perspective of our everyday lives, a day 100 centuries hence may seem remote to the point of absurdity. Yet our present day will eventually take its permanent place in the ancient history of humankind. That distant future day will come. And it could be the first day of the rest of your life."

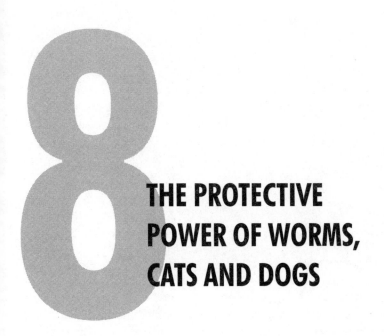

8

THE PROTECTIVE POWER OF WORMS, CATS AND DOGS

Pets prevent heart attacks

DESPITE BIG MEDICAL ADVANCES and increased awareness about the dangers of smoking and a poor diet, heart disease remains the principal cause of death. Each year, it kills more than 110,000 people in the UK, and 600,000 in the USA, and more than six million people in these two countries have associated diseases like angina.

While it's known that there are many diseases and lifestyle habits which increase the risk of heart disease, including high blood pressure, diabetes, high cholesterol, smoking and poor diet, there is increasing evidence that psychosocial factors – anxiety, stress and depression – contribute to the risk too. It has been shown, for example, that people who live alone are more likely to have heart disease. It has been found too that married people are less likely to get the disease, and that the never-married are 38 per cent more likely to die of heart disease. Those who have a wide circle of friends and those who socialize have been shown to be less prone to the disease.

Just how socializing and companionship protect against, or how the lack of them increases, vulnerability is not clear. One theory is that it is all down to emotional stress triggering a rise in adrenaline which makes blood clot more easily, thus increasing the risk of disease and heart attack. Companionship may reduce emotional stress and keep adrenaline levels down.

The beneficial effects of marriage and having a partner have been found in a large number of studies, but does that mean those with only non-human companions are doomed to have heart disease?

Not according to researchers at Purdue University, Indiana. They say similar beneficial effects can be had from another type of companion, a pet. In fact, they suggest, pet ownership may save thousands of lives, and that as many as 7 out of 10 of us could benefit.

Evidence shows that people can form strong emotion bonds with pets, particularly companion dogs. The benefits of having a pet, say the researchers, include a feeling of intimacy, entertainment, non-judgemental companionship and a reduction of social isolation. These are all qualities that are found in a human relationship where they have been shown to protect against stress, loneliness, depression and anxiety – all risk factors for heart disease.

The researchers cite data showing that pet ownership is linked to a 2–3 per cent reduction in mortality after a heart attack: "A similar level of risk reduction through additional primary prevention could potentially save 6,000 to 12,000 lives each year in the United States," they say. And if owning a pet also reduced the risk of having heart disease, as well as improving survival chances after a heart attack, even more lives would be saved.

"In a time of increasingly sophisticated medical technology, it seems ironic that something generally accepted as contributing to a better quality of life and present in nearly 50 per cent of all households, namely pet animals, has not been adequately examined for its possible role in protecting humans against the risks and consequences of coronary heart disease," say the researchers. "We propose that by positively influencing psychosocial risk factors in their owners, pets may reduce the risk of coronary heart disease and increase the likelihood of surviving a heart attack should it occur."

Taking the elevator for a natural birth

ON THE FACE OF IT there did not seem to be a rational explanation. Out of 198 pregnant women with labour difficulties admitted to the hospital, 42 improved dramatically, gave birth spontaneously and naturally, and no longer needed the caesarean section they had been about to have.

Since their arrival in the hospital, all the women had been given conventional treatment for a difficult labour, but all had failed to respond. Then, for no apparent reason, they each gave birth naturally minutes before surgery was due to be carried out. Many of them gave birth either on the way to or just inside the operating theatre, and each had a normal vaginal delivery before any attempt at a caesarean was made.

Investigations by the researchers showed that these sudden, unexpected natural births often occurred while the patients were being transferred from the labour room to the operating theatre, which are on different floors of the hospital.

None of the patients had received any medication before being taken to the operating theatre which could explain the sudden change, so the researchers at Shiraz University of Medical Sciences, Iran looked for another explanation, particularly factors that were common to the women. What they found was that all of the women who had given birth naturally had travelled to theatre in the hospital elevator.

One of the causes of a difficult pregnancy is that the foetus's head may be in an awkward position for a natural delivery, and the researchers suggest that the sudden movement of the elevator and the force of gravity may have changed the position of the foetus. That change in pressure, it's argued, gave the foetus an opportunity to move to a better position, leading to a spontaneous, normal delivery.

"The elevator can give the power to the foetus to have a rotation of the head to a more proper position for the rest of the labour," say the researchers. "We propose this possibility, that the sudden thrust of the elevator and the force of gravity had an impact on the position of the foetus and gave the foetus the opportunity to change to a better position which was proper for the rest of the vaginal delivery process."

Seaweed may prevent AIDS

GLOBAL DEATHS FROM AIDS CONTINUE their remorseless rise. The latest estimates suggest that worldwide there are now more than 40 million people living with HIV, with five million a year becoming newly infected and in excess of three million people dying of AIDS every 12 months.

With no cure and only long-term, expensive treatments that have considerable side-effects, better therapies are urgently needed, and billions of pounds are being spent trying to find cures and better treatments for HIV/AIDS. The US government alone has been funding research at the rate of $1 billion a year, and with other governments, pharmaceutical companies, universities and health services all heavily contributing too, the total amount being spent is huge.

Hundreds of compounds are being screened as potential treatments, many of them naturally occurring substances that have shown some kind of activity against the virus.

Some research suggests that as many as 30 per cent of drugs for all conditions, including the world's most famous pill, aspirin, have their roots in naturally occurring compounds. So it's possible that the next best treatments for AIDS, perhaps even a cure, may come from a natural compound. But what could it be?

According to researchers at the University of South Carolina and the South Carolina Cancer Center, and Marine Biomedical Research, Tasmania it could be algae, or seaweed.

A first step in tracking down any plant that could be the next super-drug is to look for indirect evidence which suggests that people who eat whatever it is, or drink it, or rub it on or even smoke it, have a lower or higher incidence of disease. And it just so happens that there are dramatic differences in HIV/AIDS prevalence rates between algae-eating populations in eastern Asia, including Japan and Korea, where about 0.1 per cent of adults are infected, and most of Africa, where infection rates may be 40 per cent or more.

There is one curious exception to the rule in Africa – Chad, where reports suggest a prevalence rate of only 2.6–3.6 per cent. Intriguingly, a popular local dish in Chad is spirulina, which is made from algae. There is also, say the researchers, some evidence that seaweed and spirulina extracts block a number of viruses, including herpes. Other research shows that five times the amount of HIV was required to infect cells that had been treated with spirulina extract. Another test showed that when a solution of an Asian seaweed, *wakame*, was added to HIV-infected cells for three days, all the infected cells disappeared.

The researchers say that eating algae before exposure to HIV may increase the amount of virus exposure needed for infection, and that continuing to eat algae may reduce the speed with which the virus reproduces after infection. Algae may also stimulate the immune system to resist the virus.

"Algae consumption might prevent or slow progression of HIV-infection to AIDS. These algal supplements have no known side-effects, so clinicians could combine it with conventional therapy to achieve maximum results," they say.

Worms prevent heart disease

IN THE SEARCH FOR CAUSES of disease, one of the first strategies is to look for geographic variation. If one group of people have a much higher or lower prevalence of disease, there may well be something about their environment or lifestyle that either increases or reduces the risk. Such epidemiological studies have been used to track down risk factors involved in many diseases. Sometimes the links have been suspected for a long time, occasionally the findings are unexpected and rarely connections have been found which at first sight seem to defy belief.

In their research into the causes of atherosclerosis, or hardening of the arteries, a cause of heart disease and stroke, a team at University Hadassah Medical School and Ben Gurion University, Israel found a significant geographic difference in prevalence. In areas with a high level of intestinal worm infections in humans, the risk of heart disease was lower, and the suggestion is that worms may protect against heart disease and stroke.

Atherosclerosis is a major health problem. The build-up of plaque, a fatty substance, usually affects large and medium-sized arteries and can increase to a level where it significantly reduces blood flow. Plaque can rupture, or break away, creating blood clots that cause heart attacks or strokes. Each year in the UK, heart disease kills more than 110,000 people, and there are almost 300,000 heart attacks.

Some risk factors for atherosclerosis are known, including high cholesterol and hypertension, smoking and diabetes, but the researchers say these do not fully explain the extent and severity of coronary artery disease in almost half of patients.

According to the research a link between atherosclerosis and worms, or helminthic infections, has never before been examined. Helminthic infections are generally found in poor areas and are highly prevalent in communities where sanitation is poor, with one estimate suggesting that up to a third of the world population is infected. The highest levels of infection are found in people aged over 50, the same age group who are at high risk of heart disease in the West.

The researchers say that while heart disease rates are much lower in developing countries, studies show that with Western lifestyles, disease rates go up. There is evidence from China, India and Africa that exposure to higher socio-economic status and westernization reverses the historically low risk for heart disease in those countries. They point out that westernization also brings better sanitation and reduces helminthic infections. Increased risk of atherosclerosis has been shown in men living in cities after sanitation had been improved. Moving from rural to urban areas with improved sanitation has also been shown, they say, to hasten the development of atherosclerosis in just one generation.

Just how worm infections affect heart disease risk is not clear, but one theory is that it may be down to the worms' own survival mechanism. The tiny worms evade or suppress the human immune system by producing anti-inflammatory compounds, which might also, it's suggested, have a protective effect in atherosclerosis.

"It is hypothesized that worms are protective against heart disease. Multiple lines of evidence support the notion that there is also an inverse relationship between helminthic infections and atherosclerosis and its related diseases," say the researchers. "The challenge for the future is to use that knowledge to develop better treatments."

Killer viruses are hiding in the ice

DEEP UNDER THE MELTING ICECAPS something sinister is stirring. Viruses, trapped in the ice for possibly millions of years in some cases may be about to escape. And some, like influenza A and polio, and others whose effects are unknown may be able to infect humans.

Researchers have calculated that there are at least 100,000,000,000,000,000 microbes, including fungi, bacteria and viruses, released from melting ice every year.

"Evidence supports the hypothesis that viral pathogens are preserved in glaciers, ice sheets and lake ice," they say. "Environmental ice traps and freezes viruses. It is our hypothesis that it entraps large numbers of pathogenic viruses. World health and eradication of specific pathogens could be affected by this huge reservoir. The increasingly frequent and mysterious appearance of epidemics involving new and severe human pathogens from unknown reservoirs provides a wake-up call, suggesting that traditional disease-monitoring systems lack sensitivity for detecting non-traditional diseases."

The theory of ice-bound viruses may explain why some diseases, like various strains of flu, arrive, infect and then simply disappear.

Researchers, from Oregon State University, State University of New York and Bowling Green State University say that for the majority of viruses, freezing preserves their integrity and potency. According to the report, viruses that could be trapped in the ice include polio as well as the influenza viruses. Polio viruses remain viable for long periods when they are frozen, and spread easily and rapidly in water.

Aquatic birds, which come into contact with water and ice, are a major carrier of the influenza A virus. The 1918 H1N1 flu virus was responsible for an estimated 20–40 million deaths, and the report says that variants of it have appeared in humans since 1918, separated in time by decades of absence. During those years it could be lying dormant in ice, and research is cited which shows that the virus has been found in a frozen Siberian lake.

There is also evidence of a number of other infections that have appeared and then mysteriously disappeared. The first known occurrence of a calicivirus infection, for example, occurred in 1932 when there was a sudden outbreak of a swine disease in California which was first thought to be foot and mouth disease. After 20 years the disease spread from California to other parts of the USA, but within four years it had disappeared altogether. Now it has been discovered that fish, which could have picked up the infection from water contaminated by melting ice, were the main carriers of the disease.

"The decades-long disappearances and subsequent reappearances of influenza A subtypes, in addition to their presence in Siberian lake ice, lends some circumstantial support to the hypothesis that ice serves as a reservoir for viable pathogenic viruses," say the researchers. "Control, surveillance and eradication efforts for pathogenic viruses should consider the possibility of entrapment in environmental ice."

Car travel causes heart disease

IS IT A COINCIDENCE that cases of lung and breast cancer, diabetes and heart disease all began to rise after the invention of the motor car? Not according to an Australian researcher, who has spent some time comparing rates of disease and car usage, looking for possible ways in which travelling by car might contribute to or even cause disease.

The suggestion is not that these diseases are caused by exposure to pollution, petrol or other toxins that comes with car use, but that the act of travelling without physical effort overloads the body's protective mechanisms, resulting in elevated levels of glucose and other compounds in the blood, which lead to disease.

The research, based on around 60 years of data in Australia, as well as the results of blood tests on a small number of drivers, found what is described as a marked connection between deaths due to lung cancer, diabetes and breast cancer, and travelling in a motor vehicle. According to the report, an examination of records of deaths caused by lung cancer, diabetes and breast cancer show that their incidence per 100,000 population was very small before the twentieth century and the arrival of the car. But as car use has increased, so too has the prevalence of the diseases.

After reviewing all the evidence, the report suggests the effortless travel theory. The idea is that when the body senses it is on the move, there are physical changes in the autonomic and sympathetic nervous systems which cause changes in the blood. The suggestion is that when the body perceives itself to be moving, the brain assumes that energy will be needed and makes itself ready for walking or running. But when little or no body energy is needed, because the car is doing all the work, body mechanisms start malfunctioning because the changes that have been made are not needed.

"It is contended that these changes are responsible for the development of these diseases. It is suggested that vehicle travel affects the circulatory or nervous systems which are common to the diseases," says the report.

To test the theory that driving affects blood levels of glucose and other compounds, tests were carried out on 10 men aged 19–62 at the Royal Hobart Hospital Physiology Department. Blood tests were taken before and after a 15-minute drive at speeds not exceeding 50 mph. Analysis of the results showed significant changes in levels of glucose, cholesterol and tryglycerides between the samples taken immediately after driving and those taken before – glucose levels, for example, went up by around 18 per cent.

"Blood content changes during the driving test strongly support the hypothesis that driving is the cause of heart disease," says the report. "The driving tests have revealed that physiological changes do take place as a result of driving. The author is of the opinion that these changes could be involved in many disorders, hormonal, blood and nervous conditions and may even have deleterious affects extending to the expectant mother and the unborn child."

How soft drinks prevent stomach cancer

BILLIONS HAVE BEEN SPENT in the search for better treatments for cancers. Every year, hundreds of clinical trials of new therapies begin and dozens of new drugs are tried. Sometimes there are major breakthroughs, but most of the time the new therapies bring welcome but relatively minor improvements.

Rarely, really big advances against cancer are made not with new treatments, but with the discovery of what causes the disease. Lung cancer, for example, is a very difficult malignancy to treat, but for most people relatively easy to prevent. The discovery that smoking was the principal cause has prevented millions of premature deaths.

Although the cause of most lung cancer had been staring researchers in the face for years, it took the epidemiological work by Sir Richard Doll half a century ago to establish a firm link with smoking.

Could something, which will become equally obvious with the benefit of hindsight, be responsible for other cancers?

The incidence of stomach cancer has declined dramatically in the USA and Western Europe in the last 50 years, although it is still a big problem in some parts of the world, including Japan. There are a number of potential causes, including infection with *Helicobacter pylori*, the bacteria that also causes many stomach ulcers. But infection does not explain all the cases, so what else could be involved?

According to a report by researcher Stephen Seely it is no coincidence that the decline in stomach cancer rates began at the same time that soft drinks and domestic refrigerators became popular. The theory is not that they provided direct protection against the cancer, but that they reduced use of a possible cause of the malignancy – hot drinks.

Hot water, it's suggested, may damage the stomach lining

making it more susceptible to cancer cells. Hot food does not have the same effect because much of its heat is lost in chewing before swallowing. The report points out that the 65 per cent decline in stomach cancer cases in the USA came shortly after the introduction of the fridge. A smaller decline of around 30 per cent came in the UK about 10 years later, in 1945.

There was an even more dramatic decline in Okinawa during the 27-year US administration. By 1972, when Japanese sovereignty was restored, the prevalence rate was 11.3 cases per 100,000 people, compared to the Japanese rate of 46.7.

At the same time as the domestic fridge was becoming popular, another lifestyle revolution was taking place with the huge rise in cold soft drinks consumption. In the 1930s, the average American was drinking 40 bottles a year, but by the 1970s, this had risen to 300. Over the same period, there was a threefold drop in stomach cancer rates. "A possible explanation is that it is not the soft drinks that have a prophylactic effect, but the hot drinks which they replace are carcinogenic," says the report. "Similarly, the effect of refrigerators is that they have popularized iced drinks as another alternative to hot drinks. Most peculiarities of the distribution of gastric cancer can be explained by the assumption that excessively hot water has a carcinogenic effect on gastric epithelium. The recession of gastric cancer can be correlated with the partial supplanting of hot drinks by soft drinks, iced drinks and the like."

Smoking caused rheumatoid arthritis

IN 1800, A YOUNG FRENCHMAN, Augustin Jacob Landre-Beauvais, wrote a dissertation for his medical doctorate that had a profound impact on a disease that affects around three million people across Europe. He suggested that the disease was not a type of gout, as had been thought, but a separate condition, and his thesis is now acknowledged to be the first description of rheumatoid arthritis. His work eventually led to new approaches being developed for the disease, although there is still no cure.

But was the young medical student describing an old disease that had been around for a long time and simply not been recognized, or was it a new condition?

Although rheumatoid arthritis has been extensively investigated, including studies of possible immune, genetic, infectious and hormonal factors, its cause, like the cure, remains elusive. It is not even known how long it has been around.

According to a New Jersey researcher, it may be no coincidence that the rise in cases of the disease in the UK and Europe happened relatively soon after the arrival of tobacco from the USA. The report cites evidence that the disease was suffered by ancient Americans, and when scans were taken of 3,000-year-old North American skeletal remains, scientists found signs of rheumatoid arthritis in the bones. Native Americans were known users of tobacco, so is it possible that the Elizabethan adventurers who first shipped tobacco to Britain also brought the cause of rheumatoid arthritis?

"If rheumatoid arthritis existed in New World inhabitants 3,000 to 5,000 years ago, but was diagnosed in Europe about the time when tobacco was introduced, tobacco could have an aetiological role," says the report. "The hypothesis of this paper is that there is a significant positive correlation between primary and secondary exposure to tobacco smoke and rheumatoid arthritis."

Just how it could have such an effect is not clear. It could be through inflammation, because rheumatoid arthritis is an inflammatory disease where the immune system attacks healthy tissue.

One potential stumbling block for the theory is that the disease is diagnosed more often in women, who would not have been the early smokers. One possible explanation is that women may have been affected by exposure to secondary smoke.

Tiny bugs living in the lungs cause asthma

DESPITE THE HUGE NUMBER of people with asthma – 1 in 12 adults in the UK – the exact cause of the disease is not fully understood. Although common triggers for attacks include colds and flu, dust, cigarette smoke, allergies and exercise, what makes some people prone to asthma and others not is unknown.

Research shows that almost 7 out of 10 asthmatics also have an allergy to the house dust mite and that more than 90 per cent of them have an antibody to a particular compound associated with the mites, Der P1. House dust mites are known to produce a range of potent allergens, including Der P1, which is produced in the mid-gut of the bug and helps it to digest the protein in human tissue.

The theory put forward in a research report from the University of Cardiff is that asthma in people who are sensitive to house dust mites may be caused by breathing in live dust mites, which then live for some time in the lungs. To provide themselves with food, the mites excrete Der P1m and eat tissue cells.

"We propose that asthma in house dust mite-sensitive patients may be caused by recurrent inhalation of live dust mites which are able to live for some time in the bronchioles of the lung," say the researchers. "There is some evidence that initial exposure to house dust mite allergens and in particular Der P1 can trigger sensitization to the allergen. In other words, that Der P1 may be causally linked to the origin of asthma in some individuals."

The mites eat the cells, but the loss of the cells leaves underlying tissue vulnerable to dust mite allergens which trigger sensitization. The repeated infestation provokes an allergic response of the classic asthma attack.

Just how the mites get in is not clear. But the report says it's not unreasonable to assume that if your nose is pressed into a pillow at night, mites will be inhaled from time to time, particularly as there are 20,000 or so to the cubic metre of the average mattress. During the night, we breathe in a round 5,000 litres of air, so the chances of live mites being inhaled are high. The size of the mites means that most would be deposited in the upper airways or the trachea rather than in the bronchioles. However, it's possible they could crawl deeper into the lungs.

The research report says that the presence of mites in the lungs is well known in other primates and has been also been found in birds, insects and other animals. It says that mites have also been found in human sputum. In one study, mites were found in the sputum of 17 out of 28 asthmatics.

9

HOW TO STAY ALIVE, KEEP THIN AND HAVE A BIG HEAD

Killer popcorn

CAN IT BE, IS IT really possible, that the 17 billion quarts of popcorn Americans eat each year cause cancer?

According to Jerome Blondell, a researcher from Springfield, Virginia, the sharp parts of the corn may create small cuts in the tissue of the colon as they pass through, which make it easier for cancer cells to get a hold. He says some research has given the illusion that the major causes of colon cancer have already been identified – meat, fats, alcohol, bile acids and low dietary fibre – but little attention has been given to the idea these are mere surrogates for other risk factors which are of greater importance. For instance, the benefits of dietary fibre may be due to selenium and magnesium rather than the fibre itself.

And then there's popcorn: "While popcorn seems a less likely contributor to cancer than pesticides and PCBs [polychlorinated biphenyls], it must be admitted that to date this potential dietary risk factor has been ignored," he concedes, adding: "No publications could be located in the open literature in which popcorn had been studied in relation to cancer."

He did, however, locate a report on patients with cancer of the oesophagus in northern China who were found to have 10 times the level of fragments from millet bran in the mucous of their throat when compared to a healthy control group. He says the authors of that report suggest the fragments may stimulate the spread of cancer by providing anchor points for malignant cells, in much the same way that asbestos does in the lungs.

The Chinese team also suggested that the fragment's sharp edges could cause minor lacerations and scarring during their passage down the oesophagus which could also stimulate the spread of cancer cells, helping them to get a better hold on tissue.

"The sharper fragments of popcorn kernels may be responsible for lacerations and scarring which could lead to the type of fibrosis known to be associated with colorectal cancer," says the report.

Botox makes you thinner

BOTOX, THE TOXIN THAT GAVE bacteria celebrity status, is best known for ironing out wrinkles, smoothing necks, curing excessive sweating and correcting squints. Although it is being increasingly used by doctors treating symptoms in patients with other conditions too, including multiple sclerosis, cerebral palsy, spinal cord and brain injuries, as well as stroke survivors, its cosmetic effects and its use by celebrities grab the headlines.

But is Botox now ready to take on the ultimate cosmetic challenge? Can injections of botulinium toxin reduce your weight? Could a series of 40 injections get rid of that fat tummy?

Botulinum toxin is produced by *clostridium botulinum* and works by making muscles weak. It achieves that by blocking the action of the nerves and a compound called acetylcholine which triggers the muscle into contracting. That's how it works for wrinkles, facial tics or spasms.

The theory that it could be used to tackle the overweight and obesity epidemic does have some support from experiments which have shown that blocking or cutting nerves to an area of the body can result in a loss of fat in that locality. Work on rats showed that when experimenters cut the vagus nerve, one of the longest in the body, it led to localized fat loss.

Researchers at the National University of Singapore suggest that Botox injections could work in pretty much the same way by blocking the nerves – a process they call chemodenervation – which would result in loss of fat in and around the injection sites.

"We postulate that injections of Botox into adipose tissue can result in atrophy by causing chemodenervation. As such, Botox can be injected into deposits of fat, in the buttocks, thighs or abdominal area, for cosmetic purposes," they say.

The theory is that the abdomen would be divided into a grid with 40 injection sites. Each patient would then be given one injection in each of the squares of the grid to de-nerve, and hence, de-fat, each site. The use of relatively high doses of the toxin would mean it would spread around each injection site to cover each square of the gird. When all 40 sites are injected there would thus be a uniform fat loss over the whole area.

If this body sculpturing by Botox works, there may still be a couple of downsides, as well as the trauma of the 40 injections. First, Botox effects tend to wear off over time, so more injections may be needed – the Singapore researchers say the effects could last between three months and two years.

The second downside is that the technique would probably only tackle subcutaneous fat, the fat which is just under the skin, and not the deeper visceral fat. While removing the superficial fat would probably make you look better and weigh less, it won't have much impact on health because it is visceral fat which increases the risk of heart disease, stroke, diabetes and high blood pressure. Visceral fat is processed by the liver and turned into cholesterol, and bad cholesterol narrows the arteries.

"Our procedure, if feasible, would achieve cosmetic improvement without decreasing morbidity or mortality, and patients must be counselled to embark on a regimen of diet and exercise in order to decrease visceral fat as well," say the researchers.

Defecate at night to lose weight

OBESITY HAS BECOME A GLOBAL health problem. The World Health Organization estimates that more than one billion adults are overweight, with at least 300 million obese. In the UK, one in five adults are obese and more than 30,000 deaths a year are caused by obesity and associated health conditions.

Potential solutions range from dieting, lifestyle and behaviour changes to appetite-modifying drugs and surgery to shrink the stomach. But dieting does not work for many people and nor do lifestyle changes. Other strategies can be expensive, while surgery also carries the risks that come with anaesthesia and a major operation.

Investigators are constantly trying to come up with new and more effective means of tackling the problem simply and cheaply, and researchers at Leiden University Medical Centre, the Netherlands may have hit on a novel, natural and cheap solution – defecating at night.

The basic idea is that postponing going to the toilet until night time, rather than the morning, means having to carry extra weight around for the day which will result in more calories being burnt and less fat accumulating. What's more, say the researchers, the feeling of having a full colon depresses the appetite, so even fewer calories will be eaten. And although the final clearing of the bowels late at night may boost hunger, it won't mean eating more because you will be too tired and will fall asleep.

"We postulate that applying the habit of defecating just before the usual bedtime will eventually result in body weight reduction and a lower mean body weight over time," they say. "Defecating before the usual bedtime implies conducting all your activities with a few extra ounces of luggage and, just as dragging a rucksack all the time will cost you more energy, the additional faecal cargo will cause the body to expend more energy and thus lose weight. If proven effective, this could be a costless novel approach in our fight against obesity and its harmful sequelae."

But, in a second report, doctors at Aristotle University of Thessaloniki, Greece challenge the idea, pointing out that research shows that 77 per cent of people defecate in the morning. They caution that people trying to hold things back until night time may have difficulty in doing so. In fact, they say, such behaviour may upset the body clock and lead to constipation, a known risk factor for colon cancer.

"It is important to stress that people should always respond to a defecatory urge because failure to do so causes constipation," they say. "The restraint required to counterbalance the increased tendency to discharge during the day will obviously have a negative impact on both the quality of life and the productivity of the people who would wish to follow the advice in order to lose weight, as their concentration will be focused on how to avoid defecation rather than work." They add, "Our suggestion for weight loss would be to adhere to simple methods such as a balanced Mediterranean-style diet and to encourage physical activity."

Diet every other day to lose weight and live longer

A DIET THAT NOT ONLY leads to weight loss, but that tackles disease, protects against infections and even prolongs life may no longer be just a dream. A team of doctors and scientists who have been on the diet for three years say it can have an impact on conditions as diverse as asthma and heart disease. Results from the first clinical trial of the diet show what are described as a dramatic reduction in the inflammation associated with the disease.

"We have observed improvement in a variety of disease conditions, starting within two weeks, including insulin resistance, asthma, seasonal allergies, rheumatoid arthritis, osteoarthritis, infectious diseases, periodontal disease and cardiac arrhythmias," says plastic surgeon Dr James Johnson, co-author of a report on the diet along with colleagues from Stanford and New Orleans Universities.

Described by Johnson, who lost 35 pounds in the first 11 weeks of being on the diet, as the up-day, down-day diet, it involves eating as normal on one day and then restricting calorie intake the next day by between 20 and 50 per cent.

It's claimed that for people who want to lose weight, the diet has the psychological advantage of removing permanent food deprivation. It's suggested too that people are more likely to diet for one day when they know they can eat normally the next, rather than having to cut back indefinitely. But the researchers say that alternate day calorie restriction has health-promoting effects in the absence of weight loss, and that they now have data on 500 people who have used it successfully.

"For three years we have experimented with an alternate day pattern of eating in which intake is limited to 20–50 per cent of estimated daily requirement one day followed by ad lib eating the next day. This alternate day calorie restriction appears to have health-promoting effects in the absence of weight loss," says the report. It adds, "Based on a broad range of calorie restriction studies in animals in which virtually all diseases are delayed, prevented or ameliorated by calorie restriction, we propose that this dietary pattern, with or without weight loss, will delay, prevent or improve a wide variety of human diseases in addition to the above, including multiple sclerosis, Alzheimer's disease, Parkinson's disease, atherosclerosis, and congestive heart failure."

Exactly how it works is unknown, but one theory is that food deprivation switches on a gene which triggers a reaction in the body that speeds up the processing of fat. Not only does that result in a loss of weight, but it's suggested it also impacts on levels of oxidative damage which is implicated in a large number of diseases.

Salt, the cocaine of the kitchen

IT COMES AS A FINE white powder, may be addictive and can kill, and it's in almost every kitchen and on every dining table in the world.

Most people still eat too much salt despite the fact that it has been consistently linked to high blood pressure, which in turn increases the risk of stroke, heart disease, heart failure and kidney disease.

According to Yalcin Tekol of the Erciyes University Medical Faculty, Turkey, who has not used salt at the table for more than 20 years, salt fulfils all the criteria for being classed as an addictive drug. It is, he says, addictive, because users have difficulty giving up and experience withdrawal symptoms when they try to cut down, and it is bad for the health.

"It is important to recognize the addiction-inducing propensity of salt in order to battle better with this insidious health-destructive substance," he says. "As the main culprit for developing hypertension and producing or promoting other important health problems, salt intake causes millions of deaths in the world yearly. The recognition of the addictive properties of salt will facilitate combating these health problems."

He has, he says, personal experience of withdrawal symptoms. At the beginning of his saltless period, meals seemed tasteless and he had anorexia and nausea before his body adapted to his new regime. Another signs of it being a drug, he says, is that patients with high blood pressure find it difficult to cut back despite being warned about the health consequences. Consumers also increase their levels of intake over time, another symptom associated with drug addiction. "The difficulties of salt restriction in hypertensive patients despite intense counselling campaigns seems to be the most important evidence indicating salt addiction," he says.

NB: Salt is sodium chloride and, according to the *Dietary Guidelines for Americans*, adults should consume less than one teaspoon of salt a day. Around 75 per cent of the salt we eat is added by manufacturers, and only 10 per cent is added at the table.

Why American heads are getting smaller (and the French bigger)

CAN IT BE REALLY BE true that American heads are getting smaller? According to research, there is little doubt. Hats bought in the USA have gone down in size so much, it seems, that older people with larger heads now have difficulty in finding one to fit. Also, it's suggested, visitors to Paris who care to compare the heads of young Frenchmen with those of same age American tourists will be surprised to discover that the French have obviously larger heads. Observers may also notice that the heads of American men and women are also becoming longer and narrower.

These and other facts on the diminishing size and changing shape of the heads of young Americans can, it's suggested, be explained by diet, and in particular hormones used in meat production.

Many natural and synthetic sex hormones have been used in the livestock and poultry businesses for more than half a century. Some research has suggested that these hormones can be linked to disease and physiological changes, including cancer, congenital malformations, sterility and ovarian cysts. It has been suggested in the UK, says the report, that hormonal traces in the meat of chemically treated livestock are causing British girls to mature at least three years earlier. Multiple cases of premature puberty caused by oestrogen-contaminated meat have also been seen in Puerto Rico.

Exactly how dietary hormones could result in small heads is not clear, but one theory is that they selectively help the growth process. What that means is that the build-up of hormones from the diet accelerates growth in long bones, which increase height and limb length, at a much faster rate than other bones. They may also trigger a stop in the growth of other bones.

"The general acceleration of growth caused by hormones affects long bones more than any other tissue, and it triggers inhibitors of growth during earlier stages of flat bone development. Because of that, the relative size of the skull with respect to the body is diminished. This change of body/head proportion could be accompanied by a diminution in the absolute size of the skull as well," says the report.

"Not only the size of the head, but also the shape could be influenced by intake of meat and milk from hormonally treated animals. One possibility is that the generation of young Americans may have been affected by hormonal food, which diminished their head size and changed the head shape."

The research finds considerable observational evidence for a decline in the size of American heads. It says that in American synagogues, members of older generations have larger heads than younger family members. But there is no visible difference in the size of the heads between the young and older generation of Soviet Jews who would have both grown up without hormonal food. Children of Soviet immigrants who grew up in the USA were observed to have smaller heads than their counterparts in Russia. In Israel a similar pattern emerged. Native Israelis as well as young American immigrants and tourists had smaller heads than the young immigrants from the Soviet Union, France or South America.

The report suggests that the reason why French heads are bigger is because of differences in the French and the American diet over the last 25 years, and restrictions in France on the use of hormones in the food industry.

Eating pork causes multiple sclerosis

FOR YEARS, THE WIDE GEOGRAPHIC differences in the prevalence of multiple sclerosis have baffled researchers. Most studies have shown that rates are higher closer to the north and south poles compared to places nearer the equator. In the USA, for example, the prevalence is about twice as high in North Dakota as it is in Florida, and the UK has higher rates than Spain.

Environmental factors, from the diet to the sun and vitamin D, have been investigated as possible reasons for the difference, but the cause of the disease remains elusive. Or does it? Research at the University of Ottawa and Ottawa General Hospital suggests a new culprit – pork.

In their search for a cause, the researchers reasoned that if there was a link between a dietary factor and MS, there should be similarities in the geographic distribution of the disease and the consumption of whatever the dietary factor is. In their study, the researchers looked at the relationship between consumption of total fat, beef and pork in several countries, and the prevalence rates for MS which affects around 85,000 people in the UK. Links between consumption of beef and pork and latitude were also investigated.

The study shows that there is a clear geographic link between total fat eaten and MS prevalence. The relationship between the numbers of cases of MS and pork eating was highly significant, but no such relationship was found for beef. There was also a strong link between pork consumption and latitude, but little relationship for beef. The researchers say the results are in line with reports that MS is rare in countries where pork is forbidden by religious customs, and that it has a low prevalence in countries like Brazil and Australia where beef consumption far exceeds pork consumption.

Just how eating pork might increase the risk of developing MS is not known.

One theory is that a high intake of saturated fats is to blame. But that would not explain why a link was found with pork, but not with beef. Another suggestion is that there are greater amounts of linoleic acid in pork compared to beef, but that would make pork less likely to increase risk because studies have shown that linoleic acid can reduce the severity and duration of relapses in MS.

Another possibility is that the fatty acids in pork and beef are different and may therefore have different effects on the protective sheath that surrounds and protects nerve fibres in the brain which become damaged in patients with MS. One suggestion is that the fatty acids in pork increase vulnerability to damage, while those in beef do not.

"The correlation between pork and MS prevalence is impressive enough and if it is valid, would imply that pork consumption is somehow related to the risk of developing MS," say the researchers. "We have shown that the amount of pork consumed correlates strongly with prevalence rates for MS and with latitude. The strength of the correlation is impressive enough to speculate that pork increases the risk of developing MS. The relationship between pork and MS deserves further study."

Mad flour disease

IN THE MIDDLE OF THE twentieth century, more than half the flour produced in the UK used a bleaching process to make sure it was as white as possible. Widely used in the USA, Canada and other countries too, the so-called agene method for bleaching flour also produced bread that rose and looked better. It also made more bread with less flour. But according to research at British Columbia University, it also contained a compound which may be a cause of the rise in the number of cases of neurological conditions, including Alzheimer's, Parkinson's and motor neurone disease or ALS.

The compound methionine sulphoximine (MSO) is a by-product of the process of bleaching flour with nitrogen dichloride gas. When it is mixed with unprocessed wheat flour, the gas makes it whiter by bleaching pigments and altering the wheat. Although the process was first patented in 1921 in the USA, the technique is thought to have been in use from much earlier in the century.

The researchers say that at times, especially during the Second World War, 80 per cent of flour was produced in this way in the UK, until it was superseded by superior production methods and went out of favour in the 1950s.

According to the researchers, MSO first began to attract attention with persistent reports that dogs fed high quantities of flour treated by the agene process showed symptoms of a neurological disorder known as running fits or canine hysteria, which had some features of epilepsy.

The role of MSO in disease development and progression is thought to be through its effects on antioxidants which act against oxidative stress. The researchers say there is increasing evidence pointing to oxidative stress as a key factor in the death of brain cells in a number of human neurological disorders.

MSO blocks the production of two key molecules: glutathione (GSH) and glutamine. GSH is a key antioxidant and any reduction reduces the body's antioxidant defences and may lead to increased oxidative stress. Reduction in glutamine may also result in a rise in the levels of ammonia, which has been linked to Alzheimer's disease.

The researchers say that cells in the nervous system are particularly sensitive to a decline in either GSH or glutamine, both considered essential for cell health and viability in the nervous system. They say the combined effects of a drop in levels of both compounds as a result of long-term exposure to MSO in bleached flour, may have had drastic effects on nerve cell health and survival

Not everyone who ate the flour developed disease, and the researchers suggest that co-triggers may be at work, including genetic predisposition, age and natural GSH levels.

"The history of MSO is intriguing and disturbing," say the researchers. "We propose the hypothesis that increased levels of neurodegenerative disorders in humans may have arisen due to inclusion in the diet of MSO, a by-product of the bleaching of flour. The potential for MSO, taken as part of a diet over a long period, to induce neuronal damage might be considerable, and seems to us to warrant further investigation."

Milk causes cancer

BIG LIFESTYLE CHANGES STARTED HAPPENING in Japan after the end of the Second World War.

The end of hostilities brought a new, peaceful invasion of Western influences, fads and fashions that challenged, and in some cases replaced, old traditions.

One of the biggest changes was in diet. Meat and dairy

products had not been part of the traditional Japanese diet, but the end of the war saw the start of a remarkable rise in consumption. According to researchers at the Medical University of Yamanashi, milk consumption in particular increased more than 20-fold, while the amount of meat eaten went up by 900 per cent, and the numbers of eggs increased 7-fold.

The striking increase in milk consumption has continued over the last half a century or more. In 1950, average consumption was 6.8 g/day. But by 1998, it had climbed to 135 g/day. Over the same period significant increases were also occurring in the prevalence of two diseases – testicular and prostate cancer. The increases were of the same order as those that had been seen in dairy consumption. The death rate from prostate cancer increased 25-fold in less than 50 years. Increases were also being seen, but at nowhere near the same level, in many Western countries, where there had been a smaller rise in dairy product use. The incidence of both cancers is much higher in Western countries than in Asian countries.

Could there be a link? Is it possible that dairy products were involved in the two cancers?

In their research, the Japanese team looked at the incidence and mortality rates of testicular and prostate cancers in 42 countries and compared them with differences in diet to see if there were any links with consumption of dairy products. Cheese was found to be most closely correlated with the incidence of testicular cancer in men aged 20–39, and milk to cancer of the prostate.

Another clue came from research in Denmark which showed that the incidence of testicular cancer was low in men born during the Second World War, when many foods, including dairy products, were in short supply.

In a second study, the team looked at 50 years of cancer statistics in Japan and compared them with foods eaten, including milk and dairy products, eggs, meat, fish and fishery products, cereals, fats, oils and pulses. The death rate per million of testicular cancer in Japan was 0.98 in 1947, increasing rapidly to reach a maximum rate of 3.49 around 1975, and then decreasing gradually to a low of 1.61 in 1995. The drop, say researchers, may be due to improved cancer treatments that were introduced in the 1970s. The death rate per 100,000 for prostate cancer was 0.24 in 1947, rising to 5.94 in 1995.

Just what in dairy products could be involved in cancer is not clear, but the researchers say that as well as fats, milk contains large quantities of the oestrogens. The female hormone concentration in modern dairy milk is high because the cows are almost always pregnant.

Hormones are thought to play a role in all three cancers, prostate, testicular and breast, and the researchers cite one study in East Anglia which showed that men with testicular cancer had consumed significantly more milk in adolescence than those without the disease. "It is not unreasonable to assume that the increased incidence of testicular cancer in the past 50 years in western countries is associated with the increased consumption of milk and dairy products," they say. "The increased consumption of meat, eggs, and milk and dairy products in Japan after the Second World War may be one cause of the remarkable increase in the number of deaths from prostate cancer during the same period. Milk and dairy products might have played a major role, since they contain considerable amounts of oestrogens in addition to saturated fats."

Rats spread mad cow disease to humans

RATS ARE NOT EXACTLY MAN'S best friend. They may be best known for their starring role in the Bubonic Plague, or Black Death, of the Middle Ages, but there are more than 30 other diseases associated with the rodents and their droppings, from rat-bite fever to eosinophilic meningitis, an infection of the brain.

But is it possible that they are also responsible for the spread of mad cow disease? Could the human form of the disease – variant Creutzfeld-Jakob disease or vCJD – be spread by rat droppings?

Bovine Spongiform Encephalopathy (BSE, popularly known as mad cow disease) is a progressive, degenerative, incurable and fatal disease that affects the central nervous system of cattle. Its cause is unknown, but the main theory is that it is caused by an infectious form of proteins called prions which are found in the brains and spinal cords of animals with the disease. BSE has been linked to animal feed containing material infected with scrapie, another prion disease found in sheep.

Variant Creutzfeldt-Jacob disease, the human form of the disease, also involves prions, and the conventional view is that BSE was transmitted to humans when they ate infected beef.

In their report "Are humans getting 'mad-cow disease' from eating beef, or something else?" researchers at the University of the Philippines say that there are now a number of prion diseases or transmissible spongiform encephalopathy (TSE) affecting different animals. The researchers, whose study included comparing human and animal prion proteins, say that while it is widely believed that vCJD may have been caused by consumption of infected beef, others routes are possible.

"Since rats and mice are known to be susceptible to prion disease, we propose that ingestion of infected rodent parts, possibly droppings, may be a possible mode of transmission of scrapie or BSE to humans," they say. "We propose that TSE may have been orally transmitted to humans who had unknowingly ingested matter, possibly droppings, from TSE-infected rats or mice." They add, "The practice of including animal carcasses in animal feed (including pet food) is undoubtedly increasing the exposure of rodents to scrapie, BSE, and other TSE. The increased likelihood of transmitting TSE to humans may be an unintended consequence of this practice."

10

TV, HIGH HEELS AND OTHER CAUSES OF ILLNESS

How a prescription drug increased depression in children

FOR UNKNOWN REASONS, THE NUMBER of children with severe depression or bipolar disorder has increased dramatically over the last 30 years. It's not only affecting more and more children, it is also being diagnosed at a much earlier age. The most recent US data show that the average age at onset is now four and a half years earlier than it used to be. Research also shows that among patients who are now aged over 45, only a few had symptoms before the age of 20, but more than half the patients who are aged 25–45 had symptoms at an early age. Even more striking, almost all of those who are now 25 had the illness by the time they were 20.

Bipolar disorder, also known as manic-depressive illness, is a brain disorder that causes unusual fluctuations in mood, energy and ability to function. Symptoms are severe and can result in damaged relationships, poor job or school performance and in some cases suicide, so it is important to find out why the incidence of the disease is increasing.

A number of possible reasons for the rise have been suggested, including increased awareness and changes in diagnosis, but none fully explains what has been happening.

There is a heavy genetic loading with the disease, which suggests that because people with severe depression are less likely to mate and have children, the number of cases should be going down rather than up.

So just what could explain the increase is not clear, but researchers at the University of Louisville suggest that the rise may be linked to the introduction of lithium, the first mood-stabilizing medication approved by the US Food and Drug Administration for the treatment of mania. They say that the current increase in bipolar illness began one generation after the introduction of the drug.

Lithium is still prescribed and is a very effective drug for controlling symptoms. The theory put forward by the researchers is that the widespread use of lithium beginning in the 1970s resulted in health improvements that led to significant changes in the lifestyles of people with the disease. In others words, the health of many patients improved so much that it led to an increased likelihood of mating and reproduction. Patients would also have spent more time in the community than before, increasing the chances of social contact. If fertility increased, more children would have been born to patients, with a greater likelihood of inheriting genes associated with the condition. Hence the rise in cases now being diagnosed.

Bipolar illness is a genetic condition whose symptoms worsen with successive generations, so the children of the first generation of lithium-treated patients would be expected to have earlier age of onset and a generally more severe course of illness. And that is what is now being seen.

"Now, 35 years after lithium was approved, we might be seeing the pre-pubertal grandchildren of that first lithium-treated generation, who have earlier age of onset of their disorder than their parents," says the report. "These pharmacological and social changes may have all conspired to increase reproductive success of bipolar subjects, giving rise to a new generation of bipolar patients with earlier onset and more severe manifestation of their disorder," say the researchers.

MS and the domestic cat

ALTHOUGH IT AFFECTS MORE THAN 85,000 men and women in the UK, and five times as many in the USA, multiple sclerosis remains a mystery, with no known definite cause or cure.

The most common disabling disease of the central nervous system affecting young adults, it's now thought to be an autoimmune disease – the immune system turns on the body's own tissue and attacks it. In MS, it attacks the myelin sheath which protects the nerves in the central nervous system, disrupting the way messages are carried to and from the brain.

There may be a genetic element to the disease, and there will also be environmental triggers. MS is also known to occur more frequently in areas that are furthest from the equator, so sunshine and vitamin D have been implicated. Viruses, bacteria and other microbes are under suspicion too, and more than a dozen, including measles, herpes and Chlamydia pneumonia, have been investigated, but with no firm conclusions.

Whatever is suggested as a potential cause has to fit in with a series of curious facts about the disease. As well as the variation in rates with distance from the equator, there is a higher incidence in people of European ancestry, in women and in people living in urban areas.

One possible answer, according to research at the School of Veterinary Studies in Murdoch, Australia, is the domestic cat. Not only would it explain the prevalence variations, there is also a virus found in cats that just might be the mechanism by which the disease is transferred. The report says it may explain the epidemiology of MS better than anything previously proposed. The theory is that as many as 7 per cent of domestic cats have a condition similar to MS, and that it can be passed to children under 15 where it remains dormant, waiting to be triggered by an event like physical or emotional stress later in life.

According to the researchers, the cat theory passes all the tests. MS is primarily a disease of people with European ancestry and they are the most likely to share their homes with a cat. The latitude differences fit in with the lower level of cat keeping around the equator and the tendency to handle pets less often in tropical climates, thus reducing the possibility of transmission of the virus. Women may also be more at risk because they cuddle cats more than men do. The rural/urban difference is explained by the fact that in rural areas, where MS is less common, cats are more likely to live outdoors.

The suggestion is that many more people have the virus that causes MS than have the disease itself, because a trigger is needed to make it active. That trigger may be a genetic vulnerability or stress. It is significant, according to the research, that most people first get the clinical symptoms around the age of 30 years when work, family and money stress levels are at their highest.

"The present hypothesis that persistent paramyxovirus present in cat central nervous tissue is transmissible to humans and is responsible for MS can be used to explain many of the epidemiological aspects of the human disease. It has been stated several times that MS may be due to some aspect of the lifestyle of people of European origin that is different to that of other races. In poliomyelitis it was hygiene, perhaps in MS it is the cat."

Soap causes heart disease

MILLIONS OF PEOPLE AROUND the world have changed their lifestyle in the belief that poor diet, high cholesterol, smoking and lack of exercise cause furring of the arteries. High dietary levels of bad cholesterol and low amounts of antioxidants in particular are blamed for hardening of the arteries or arteriosclerosis, a principal cause of heart disease and stroke.

But what if there was another villain that had so far escaped attention? Is it purely a coincidence that the rise in heart disease has coincided with the global increase in the use of soap? Could it be that every time we wash our hands we are increasing the risk of heart disease?

According to Baton Rouge researcher Robert Cane, soap is not only involved in heart disease, but other conditions too, including skin problems from poison ivy, and he cites a number of cases of people who have regained good health after they stopped using soap. Medical literature, he says, abounds with references to dietary intakes of fats and cholesterol, but the concept that they are solely to blame has inconsistencies which cannot be easily explained. Why is it, he asks, that Eskimos and desert nomads don't get the disease even though a large part of their diet is made up of fats and cholesterol? Cane says any potential cause should be able to account for anomalies like that. And that's where soap comes in.

Soap, as he points out, is a relatively recent addition to human lifestyle, with large-scale commercial production starting in the middle of the nineteenth century. Over the years, the use of soap has increased dramatically. In the early days, and before heart disease was so prevalent, it was a luxury and might have been used once a month, but in more recent times it's used many times a day.

Such chronic use, it's suggested, has interfered with the skin's natural protective processes, in particular the production of sebum in the sebaceous glands, and perspiration from the sweat glands. These natural secretions, it's argued, coat the skin and hair with protective inorganic and organic molecules. In their role of protecting the skin, the glands are constantly resupplying the skin with a new covering of cholesterol, cholesterol esters, fatty acids and triglycerides. Each time we wash with soap, the gland re-coats the skin with cholesterol. So the more we wash, the greater the amount of fat deposited on the skin. According to the second part of the theory, these larger amounts of cholesterol then get into the blood, building up plaque and eventually damaging the walls of arteries and restricting blood flow. "It is postulated that the regular use of soap causes atherosclerotic plaque."

There is no problem with washing the body with water. In fact, Cane suggests, it is possible to get used to not using soap very quickly, and that after three or four days the body skin no longer feels greasy and dirty. "In no time at all there is a greater feeling of robust wholesome good health which is difficult to explain."

Autism and city life

FOR MORE THAN HALF A CENTURY, the cause of autism has eluded investigators around the world. It has been linked to genes, unknown viruses, childhood vaccines, weakened immune systems, maternal depression, environmental toxins and pollutants, and to diet.

While the search for a cause, which would at least increase the chances of better treatments if not a cure, is still ongoing, the number of children with the condition has been rocketing. Since the early 1980s, the incidence has risen 10-fold, and while improved diagnosis may explain some of that rise, it does not account for most of it.

Genes have been the number 1 suspect, but not one has been found, and some researchers now question the importance of any genetic effect. If, they argue, genes are responsible, and since autism brings no evolutionary advantage, why has the gene and the condition not disappeared? Autistic people are less likely to marry and have children, so over time there should be a drop, not a rise, in numbers.

"Despite the fact that autism is considered to be one of the most genetic of all neurodevelopmental disorders, and despite the fact that those with autism rarely marry and pass on their genes, there has been a dramatic increase in autism in all industrialized nations over the past 25 years. The rise in autism is paradoxical in that autism should either be stable or even declining," says Texas-based researcher, Fred Previc. He suggests that prenatal factors may be important in the development of the condition and may explain findings that have been previously put down to genes. The fact that twins are more likely to both have autism may be due to what happens to the mother-to-be after conception, rather than to genes.

One candidate, it's suggested, is dopamine, which is involved in brain processes that control movement, emotional response and the ability to experience pleasure and pain. Previc says that people with autism suffer severe social and communicative deficits and delays, including reduced social skills, difficulty in judging others' expressions and intent, and repetitive behaviours. All of these, he says, can be traced back to over-production of dopamine. He cites animal studies that show that when dopamine levels go up, there is reduced social play, increased social isolation and increased repetitive behaviours. Excessive dopamine stimulation also leads to a fixation on inanimate objects, another trait found in people with autism. He says there is also evidence that stimulant drugs that boost dopamine activity in the brain tend to make autistic symptoms worse.

But if dopamine is implicated, what could be responsible for a prenatal rise in levels that would be needed to trigger such an increase in cases over such a relatively brief period of time?

According to the research report, a number of societal changes could have fuelled the rise in levels of the brain chemical, including increased maternal age, city living and the rise in the proportion of working women and the effects of this on stress levels. Stress, says the report, is associated with higher levels of dopamine. It points out that there are higher rates of autism in urban areas, which also have higher stress levels due to a number of factors, including close-quarters city living, overpopulation, sleep deprivation, pollution and traffic. Stress caused by the rising number of relationship breakdowns may be implicated too, while increased maternal age may be associated with heightened dopamine activity because the protective effects of oestrogen decline with age.

"The rising incidence of autism is mainly due to pre-natal, elevated dopamine levels," says the report. "Chronically high maternal levels of dopamine caused by the pressures of increasingly urbanized societies and by changing maternal demographics such as increased workforce participation, educational achievement level, and age at first birth, may be especially significant contributors to the recent autism rise."

Power lines cause depression

DEPRESSION IS ONE OF THE fastest-growing health problems. Rates have been rising relentlessly in almost every country for no clear reason. Stresses of modern life, declines in the family and its support systems, the availability of new drugs and improvements in diagnosis have all been suggested, and so too have genes, hormonal changes, seasonal light variations and diet.

Another possibility that until now has been largely overlooked is overhead power lines. They fit the bill in at least one respect in that their arrival and spread happened during the same period as the rise and spread of depression. And like patients with depression, the power lines are pretty much everywhere. But is there a causal link?

According to a researcher at Bristol University, there is, and power lines could be responsible annually for 9,000 excess cases of depression in adults, and 60 cases of suicide in the UK alone. On top of that, power lines may be responsible for 200–400 cases of lung cancer, 2,000–3,000 cases of other illnesses and 2–6 cases of childhood leukaemia.

The research centres on the effects of both electric and magnetic fields around high-voltage power lines in the UK. It's suggested that power frequency magnetic fields may have an effect on depression through their action on melatonin, the hormone secreted by the pineal gland in the brain, which plays a key role in regulating the circadian rhythm. Research has shown that some people with depression can be helped by taking melatonin supplements, while other studies suggest that magnetic fields are associated with changes in the way the pineal gland works, reducing the amounts of melatonin produced. It's suggested that such a theory may also explain an increase in hospital admissions for depression which have been reported during geomagnetic storms.

"Overall, the evidence confirms the potential for an association between power frequency magnetic fields and both depression and suicide," says the report. On lung cancer, it says there is evidence indicating that the risk is associated with air pollution as well as smoking. The theory implicating power lines in cancer is that when they are inhaled, electrically-charged aerosol particles have a higher chance of being deposited in the lung compared with uncharged aerosols. All airborne particles, including charcoals, bacteria, viruses and pollens, are susceptible to charging by the power lines, and as a result, it's suggested, acute respiratory and cardiovascular illness, including aggravated asthma and allergies, could all occur with higher frequency near high-voltage power lines. It is estimated that in total 2,000–3,000 excess cases of pollution-related illness could occur annually near power lines in the UK alone.

"The hypothesis is put forward that exposure to power line electric and magnetic fields results in increased risk of a range of illnesses, both cancer and non-cancer, in both adults and children," says the report. "If, as is hypothesized, several thousand excess cases of ill health occur each year near high-voltage power lines in the UK, then clearly this would be of serious public health concern. The implications warrant urgent consideration by scientists and by health and regulatory bodies."

Heeled shoes cause schizophrenia

SHOEMAKERS WHO INTRODUCED THE FIRST heeled footwear may have a lot to answer for. Not only did they start a trend which led to generations of women being condemned to wearing fashionable stiletto heels, they could also be responsible for the increasing number of cases of schizophrenia.

A link between the two may seem unlikely, but researcher Jarl Flensmark reckons the case is pretty overwhelming. In fact, "I suggest that there is an association between the use of heeled footwear and schizophrenia. I have not been able to find any contradictory data. After heeled shoes are introduced into a population, the first cases of schizophrenia appear," he says.

The theory is that heeled footwear began to be used more than 1,000 years ago and may have led to the first cases of schizophrenia and the establishment of the first mental hospitals. According to the research, as industrialization of shoe production spread eastwards from North America to England and Germany, and then to the rest of Western Europe, there was a remarkable rise in the number of schizophrenia cases. Although much research has been carried out into schizophrenia, the exact cause remains unknown, and many theories have been put forward. It has been said to be wholly or partly genetic, that unknown environmental factors are to blame, that early infections are involved and that the season of birth and temperature at conception or birth could be implicated.

The heel theory has its origins in the demise of the flat-footed moccasin and the rise of the elevated shoe heel. Although upright walking probably started around 10 million years ago, the first type of shoe came much later and was probably a basic flat leather platform or wraparound. According to the research, the oldest heeled shoe known to man comes from Mesopotamia, which, coincidence or not, is exactly the same area where the first institutions dealing with mental disorders appeared, in Baghdad (AD 750) and Cairo (873).

There are other links or coincidences too, according to the research. Schizophrenia appears to have been initially more prevalent in the upper classes, who would have been the first to begin wearing the newly fashionable heels. In England the heeled shoe came into use from the beginning of the seventeenth century, and was followed by a large increases in the number of cases of mental illness.

Another piece of evidence put forward is that Native Americans, who wear flat moccasins, have a relatively low frequency of schizophrenia, and regions with heavy rainfall, where heeled shoes are more common, have higher rates of the disease. Prevalence rates in a rural area in western Ireland with a high rainfall are more than seven times the rate found in drier Dublin.

But if all these are genuine links and not coincidences, what could be the mechanism? How could wearing heels trigger the development of mental illness? The answer, it seems, is simple. When we walk, the movement stimulates receptors in the lower extremities which increase activity in brain cells. But wearing heeled shoes weakens the lengthening contractions in the lower leg and foot, so the receptors are stimulated less. This drop in stimulation leads to changes in the dopamine system in the brain. That fits neatly with the theory that the brains of patients with schizophrenia produce more dopamine than healthy brains. It also tallies, says the report, with the finding that electrical stimulation of parts of the brain can improve functioning in patients with schizophrenia.

Fluoride makes teeth crooked

ALTHOUGH LONG ADDED TO WATER supplies and toothpastes as a way of preventing tooth decay, fluoride has not been without its critics. While considerable research points to its beneficial effects on teeth health, excessive amounts have been linked to a yellowing of teeth, white spots and pitting or mottling of the tooth enamel. More controversially, there have been claims of links with osteoporosis.

According to Philip Sutton, a researcher in Australia, it may also be responsible for something else – orthodontic problems. It's suggested that fluoride damages the developing bone whose job is to hold the teeth in place, resulting in overcrowding, crooked teeth and other dental problems.

For teeth to be straight and in their correct position, there needs to be normal development of the alveolar bone in which the teeth are anchored. One of the requirements for a healthy alveolar, like any other bone, is that two types of cell, the osteoblasts and the osteocytes, one which makes new tissue and the other which takes away the old, must work together and in balance. The suggestion is that fluoride is toxic to these cells. If the bone develops a problem like fluorosis, which is caused by too much fluoride, it can interfere with bone growth. If the bone cannot achieve its full potential shape and size, overcrowding of teeth may be the result.

The report says that severe fluorosis deformities have been seen in people, including children under 10, who habitually drink water which contains as little as 3.5 mg/l fluoride. It also cites reports of marked increases in the fluoride level in the environment, including water, food and the atmosphere, adding to the amounts of fluoride being ingested.

"It is suggested that orthodontic problems may arise as a result of increased fluoride ingestion, mainly through the fluoridation of drinking water," says the report. "When the fluoride intake from all sources is high enough to affect developing teeth, indicated by the development of dental fluorosis in some children, it is probable that the osteoblasts and the osteocytes will also be affected, in children of all ages, disrupting the normal processes of bone turnover, especially in the alveolar bone supporting the teeth."

Rain causes blood clots

WHEN SPECIALISTS ANALYSED THE SCANS and case notes of their patients, they made a curious discovery. Comparison of admissions dates with the weather on those days showed that there was a much greater likelihood of them being admitted when it had been raining or when vapour pressure, a measure of humidity, was higher.

The patients had each been admitted for pulmonary embolism, a condition where an artery in the lung becomes blocked, usually by one or more blood clots that have travelled from another part of the body, often the calf. It is a significant cause of hospital deaths, particularly among people who have had surgery, and is also an increasing threat to passengers travelling on long-distance air flights.

What has perplexed researchers for some time is that although in many cases there are known causes, there also appear to be seasonal variations in the incidence of thrombosis and pulmonary embolism. A general view has been that cold weather, which makes blood flow more sluggish, or higher air pressure, which could squeeze blood vessels reducing blood flow, may be to blame.

Researchers at Royal Surrey County Hospital, Guildford say

emergency departments find it impossible to predict how many cases of pulmonary embolism will occur on any one day. There may be many on one day, but then none for several days or even weeks. The rumour in emergency departments, they say, is that embolisms tend to occur more often when the weather is bad or when it rains.

When patients are admitted with a suspected embolism, it is routine practice for a nuclear medicine lung scan to be taken. So to see if there was any substance to the rumour, the Surrey team looked at more than 300 scans taken over a six-year period. The monthly total of scans was then compared with monthly climate data recorded at a weather station near the hospital. Measurements taken included temperature, humidity, vapour pressure, air pressure and rainfall.

The surprising results show that although there were rapid air pressure changes in the winter months, this did not have an effect on the incidence of pulmonary embolism admissions, and neither did humidity or temperature. But there was a link with both vapour pressure and rainfall. What rain and water vapour have in common is that they both put droplets of moisture into the air. Water vapour gets into the atmosphere by evaporation of water from oceans, lakes, wet roads and vegetation.

Could it be that there is something in the moisture that is responsible for the increased risk on wet days? According to the Surrey theory, pollutants trapped in the moisture may be to blame. When they are inhaled by people at risk, the particles get into the lungs and may aid the clotting process.

"It is postulated that pollutants such as diesel or aeroplane exhaust particles, trapped in windborne vapour droplets are inhaled by people exposed to this pollution, either by staying in polluted areas or downwind from them," say the researchers. "These polluted vapour droplets are absorbed by the lung and hasten coagulation cascades in the blood. This may lead to thrombosis and increased pulmonary embolism incidence under high vapour pressure conditions. With combined factors such as pre-existing ill health or immobility on long flights, the risk of thrombosis and consequent embolism might increase substantially."

Climate change caused diabetes

AROUND 14,000 YEARS AGO, northern Europe became much colder. Life on earth had been getting warmer with the retreat of the Ice Age, and plants and wildlife had been slowly moving north to the British Isles, northern Europe and beyond. But then the ice returned and the mini-Ice Age, the Younger Dryas, came and lasted for more than 1,500 years. It was so cold that there were glaciers in southern Ireland and as far south as Wiltshire, while Glasgow was buried beneath a vast ice cap.

This sudden temperature change had a devastating effect on fledgling wildlife and plants. It also had a devastating effect on humans who had begun moving into the new, warmer and newly fertile areas. Research suggests that the ancient population of northern Europe, which had peaked 14,000 years ago, dramatically declined as the mini-Ice Age set in. The populations in northern and western Europe plunged to their lowest levels during the Younger Dryas, because people either died or migrated south to warmer areas. They did not start recovering until conditions warmed up again around 11,000 years ago.

Because the drop in temperature was so dramatic, and because it came so suddenly, there would, in evolutionary terms, have been huge selection pressure for survival. In other words, those who had a gene or trait that gave them an edge in such extreme cold would have been more likely to survive, mate and produce offspring with the same genetic advantage. And that ancient genetic advantage should still be around. But what is it? According to researchers at Mount Sinai School of Medicine, New York and the University of Toronto, what emerged to protect humans was type 1 diabetes. Also know as insulin-dependent or juvenile diabetes, it occurs when the body makes little or no insulin, and usually commences early in life. Its cause is unknown, although a combination of inherited genes and environmental factors have been thought likely. The hormone insulin is vital because without it, blood-sugar levels can rise to dangerous levels.

One of the baffling facts about type 1 diabetes is that the worldwide distribution of cases is very uneven. There is a much higher prevalence in northern Europe, but it is relatively rare in Africa and Asia. Some research has also shown diabetes is first diagnosed more frequently in the winter.

"These intriguing observations raise the possibility that the cold may activate or up-regulate one or more metabolic pathways involved in the genesis of type 1 diabetes, not unlike seen in cold-tolerant animals," say the researchers. They suggest that the increased levels of glucose and other sugars in the blood may be designed to work like antifreeze in the blood, to lower the freezing point of body fluids and prevent the formation of damaging ice crystals in cells, and improve survival in extreme cold.

As an adaptation, type 1 diabetes might have worked because in those days life was short – around 25 years – and there were much greater threats. Specific traits would therefore have been selected for short-term rather than longer-term protection. But now that we expect to live much longer, diabetes has changed from carrying a survival advantage to becoming a disease.

"This cryoprotective adaptation would have protected ancestral northern Europeans from the effects of suddenly increasingly colder climates such as those believed to have arisen around 14,000 years ago and culminating in the Younger Dryas. When life expectancy was short, factors predisposing to type 1 diabetes provided a survival advantage," say the researchers. "Our hypothesis, that type 1 diabetes arose as a cryo-protective adaptation to cold environments, is compelling since it not only explains the unique prevalence of this condition in certain populations, but it is yet another example by which we have been, and continue to be, shaped by the environments in which we live."

TV shows cause dementia

OVER THE LAST HALF-CENTURY the number of people watching television has increased dramatically. During the same period, cases of dementia have also risen at an alarming rate. Coincidence, or could there be a link? After all, most people now being diagnosed with dementia will have watched television for several hours a day for much of their lives.

There have been many claims that magnetic fields, radiation and other effects of TV electronics may be hazardous to health, but this time the danger is not the equipment but the content of TV shows, and their psychological and mental effects.

Dementia is an increasing health problem affecting around 1 in 20 people aged over 65, and 1 in 5 over 80. Alzheimer's is the most common form, and so far no single factor has been identified as a cause of the disease. Age, genetic inheritance, environmental factors, diet and overall general health are among the factors that have been looked at.

According to research at Tel-Aviv University, Israel there are two problems with television that raise suspicions of a link with dementia. First, it is passive and often not very intellectually challenging; and second, many of the events it covers are stressful. Both of these effects, it's suggested, could contribute to the development of dementia.

Some research has shown that the risk of dementia is lower among higher educated people and in those involved in stimulating jobs or activities. One interpretation of these findings is that there is a "use it or lose it" theory about the brain and dementia.

In other words, those who are mentally active and use more of their brain cells are less affected or more slowly affected by the ageing process, and therefore less likely to develop the disease. Cases of dementia among Talmudic scholars in Israel, for example, are very rare.

In contrast, TV viewing is a passive activity, with little intellectual challenge, and it is one to which most elderly people have been exposed for most of their lives.

TV is also stressful. According to the researchers, by the time an American child leaves primary school, he or she will have seen 8,000 murders and 100,000 violent acts on television. The rapid increase in 24-hour news coverage means that many more stressful events, including national disasters, wars and terrorism, get far more coverage and are watched by more people.

According to the research, the stress generated by TV exposure to sad or frightening life events is stronger than other media because of the visual, real-life element and because there is no easy way for the viewer to relieve the tension. Such stress, it's suggested, affects neurones in the hippocampus, the brain region involved in memory. Similar damage is seen in brains affected by Alzheimer's.

The researchers recommend that when patients with dementia first present, details about their TV watching habits should be added to their case notes: "Considering that many individuals have by now been watching television for several decades, not infrequently at an average rate of four or more hours daily, it is possible that cumulative, stress-derived damage may magnify the risk of a dementia process in such long-term, habitual viewers," say the researchers.

Stress can seriously damage your teeth

ON THEIR LATEST ANNUAL VISIT to the Central Pacific island of Banaba, dentists made an odd discovery. During six previous trips, only 14 cases of acute dental caries were found among the 635 adults who were treated, a rate of 2.2 per cent. But during this latest trip, the number needing treatment had risen to 44 and the prevalence rate of dental disease in the population had increased almost 10-fold to 19.7 per cent. There had been no apparent change to diet or lifestyle and no marked change in the age profile, so what was responsible?

Investigations revealed that three months before the latest visit, the islanders had been told that the deposits of phosphate rock there were almost exhausted, and that the men employed in the phosphate industry would lose their jobs and be returned to the islands from where they had originally come. The researchers say that the move was accepted more easily and calmly by the women and younger unmarried men than the older men, many of whom had lived on the island for some years and had become accustomed to the considerable benefits of living and working there.

These differences in attitudes were reflected in the prevalence of acute caries. In men aged 35 and over, those who were the most stressed by the move, the prevalence was 39 per cent, far higher than the rates in women and younger men.

Further investigations revealed links between stress and acute caries. One study found that people who were being treated for depression had more caries, while a small study during routine semi-annual dental examinations of adults in a dental practice in Melbourne showed that acute dental caries were found in six adults and in five cases they had been through a period of severe mental stress. A much larger study followed involving 1,339 patients, and the results were remarkably similar. In both cases the association between stress and acute dental caries was statistically highly significant.

Just how stress could have such an effect is not clear, but one theory is that the immune system is involved. Some research shows that in depressed and stressed patients, natural killer cell activity is lower than it should be, and therefore less likely to mount a robust attack on bacteria causing tooth decay.

"It now appears that the onset of acute dental caries could be due to the failure of the immune system," say the researchers. "The data from these Micronesian and Polynesian races which usually have a very relaxed attitude to life are of interest because they show that the stress and acute dental caries relationship is not confined to people of European stock but may be present in all racial groups."

Gloves cause asthma

IT SOUNDS UNBELIEVABLE, BUT COULD the caring hands that first hold newborn babies be the source of the worldwide epidemic of asthma? Or is it just a coincidence that the global explosion in numbers of cases of asthma, allergies and eczema has come at the same time as a huge increase in powdered latex glove wearing among midwives, nurses and doctors?

According to researcher Jennifer Worth, one in five children now have asthma or eczema in childhood, and many babies seem to be either born with one or both, or to develop them within a very few days of birth.

Despite huge investment in research, no one has been able to explain why these diseases in childhood have increased so much, although many hundreds of potential culprits have been investigated, including house dust mite, cow's milk, wheat, pollen and pets.

But until now, no one has pointed the finger at latex gloves. In fact, says the research report, in more than 700 papers on latex allergy examined, not one mentions neonatal exposure to latex. Allergy to latex is seen almost exclusively as an occupational disease in adults.

Natural latex rubber comes from *Hevea brasiliensis* and contains many components, some of which are powerful allergens. Although surgical gloves made from rubber have been used for almost a century, they were originally made more simply, says the report. The process involved boiling the latex at high temperatures, and the heat destroyed most of the natural proteins which led to allergies. The gloves were supplied with no powder, and they were largely made in the UK and Europe. During the 1970s, shortly before the steep rise in asthma and allergy cases, manufacturing techniques changed. Gloves became cheap, disposable and pre-powdered, and chemicals were added to the raw latex to speed up the manufacturing process. Many of these chemicals, says the report, are not known because of patent protection.

Babies should be exposed as little as possible to contact allergens and chemicals, and yet, at the very moment of birth, babies born in delivery rooms are exposed to latex and chemicals through contact with pre-powdered latex gloves worn by midwives and doctors, it says. The chemicals also get into the air, and a delivery room is likely to contain latex-bound starch powder which, says the report, will be inhaled by the baby with its first breaths. That contact, it's suggested, may be the sensitizing event that leads to later allergic reactions and asthma.

"The evidence is in keeping with the hypothesis that neonatal exposure to latex from gloves worn at the time of delivery may be a significant sensitizing event," says the report. "Pre-powdered latex gloves have been in use for about 35 years. A whole generation has been exposed to them at birth, possibly sensitizing many children."

EXPLODING KIDNEYS, TOXIC GUITARS, AND MUCH MORE ...

BUT THAT, of course is not it.

There's more, much more, to come from the legion of scientists, physicians, researchers and enthusiasts whose unfettered original thinking continues to tackle just about anything and everything.

The sun never sets on *Medical Hypotheses*, and at this very moment someone somewhere in the world will be working in a laboratory, office, study or garden shed, honing a new theory and putting the final touches to a paper for the pages of the journal.

Which ones will be published and which will be the next blockbuster?

Well, there's the forthcoming revelation that your kidneys might explode during long-haul flights. Increased air pressure may, it seems, lead to spontaneous rupture of part of the kidney.

And there's the theory that guitar players are a health hazard. Not so much because of the loudness of the music, but as a result of nickel released from strumming the guitar strings. According to this theory, vigorous guitar players are surrounded by a near-invisible halo of nickel dust that could be responsible for high rates of asthma.

Then there are the theories that sexual orientation is determined by the foetus's immune system, that the appendix is really part of the brain and that prawns cause colon cancer. There's also the proposal that men who have the misfortune to lose one testicle may become better athletes because of the hormonal changes that result from such a loss.

Researchers have also delved into the origins and purpose of the foreskin, solved some of the mysteries of sleep, found the evolutionary reason why women suffer pain during childbirth and explained why people with dementia can still remember their favourite tunes.

And then there's a cure for AIDS ... but that's another story.

REFERENCES

Short-sighted people are more intelligent

M. W. M. Mak, T. S. Kwan, K. H. Cheng, R. T. F. Chan and S. L. Ho, "Myopia as a latent phenotype of a pleiotropic gene positively selected for facilitating neurocognitive development, and the effects of environmental factors in its expression", Volume 66, pp. 1209–15.

Revelations always happen on mountains

S. Arzy, M. Idel, T. Landis and O. Blanke, "Why revelations have occurred on mountains. Linking mystical experiences and cognitive neuroscience", Volume 65, pp. 841–5.

Fat people *really* are more jolly

K. A. Oinonen, and D. Mazmanian, "Does body fat protect against negative moods in women?", Volume 57, pp. 387–8.

Nightmares can kill you

R. B. Melles and B. Katz, "Night terrors and sudden unexplained nocturnal death", Volume 26, pp. 149–54.

Birthmarks are proof of reincarnation

I. Stevenson, "The phenomenon of claimed memories of previous lives: possible interpretations and importance", Volume 54, pp. 652–9.

Global warming reduces fertility

H. Fisch, H. F. Andrews, K. S. Fisch, R. Golden, G. Liberson and C. A. Olsson, "The relationship of long-term global temperature change and human fertility", Volume 61, pp. 21–8.

Showers are bad for the brain

R. J. F. Elsner, and J. G. Spangler, "Neurotoxicity of inhaled manganese: Public health danger in the shower?", Volume 65, pp. 607–16.

Small people can save the world

T. T. Samaras and L. H. Storms, "Secular growth and its harmful ramifications", Volume 58, pp. 93–112.

The date you will die can be calculated

S. Sri Kantha, "Total immediate ancestral longevity (TIAL) score as a longevity indicator: an analysis on Einstein and three of his scientist peers", Volume 56, pp. 519–22.

Jet lag triggers mental illness

G. Katz, R. Durst, Y. Zislin, Y. Barel and H. Y. Knobler, "Psychiatric aspects of jet lag: review and hypothesis", Volume 56, pp. 20–23.

Why humans are not furry

J. R. Harris, "Parental selection: A third selection process in the evolution of human hairlessness and skin colour", Volume 66, pp. 1053–9.

The purpose of ear wax

M. J. B. Verhaegen, "The aquatic ape theory and some common diseases", Volume 24, pp. 293–9.

Hearing voices could save your life

R. S. Bobrow, "Paranormal phenomena in the medical literature sufficient smoke to warrant a search for fire", Volume 60, pp. 864–8.

The reason for chins

I. Ichim, J. Kieser and M. Swain, "Tongue contractions during speech may have led to the development of the bony geometry of the chin following the evolution of human language – A mechanobiological hypothesis for the development of the human chin", Volume 69, pp. 20–24.

Humour increases survival

N. E. Howe, "The origin of humour", Volume 59, pp. 252–4.

Babies suck to avoid asthma

D. M. T. Fessler and E. T. Abrams, "Infant mouthing behaviour: the immunocalibration hypothesis", Volume 63, pp. 925–32.

Beer bellies protect men in old age

P. Vardi and O. Pinhas-Hamiel, "The young hunter hypothesis: age-related weight gain – a tribute to the thrifty theories", Volume 55, pp. 521–3.

Why winter swimmers don't shiver

T. M. and M. T. Kolettis, "Winter swimming: healthy or hazardous? Evidence and hypotheses", Volume 61, pp. 654–6.

Finger lengths predict disease

J. T. Manning and P. E. Bundred, "The ratio of 2nd to 4th digit length: A new predictor of disease predisposition?", Volume 54, pp. 855–7.

Arthritis is the price of having healthy ancestors

J. L. Mobley, "Is rheumatoid arthritis a consequence of natural selection for enhanced tuberculosis resistance?", Volume 62, pp. 839–43.

Feeling disgusted is healthy

M. Rubio-Godoy, R. Aunger and V. Curtis, "Serotonin – A link between disgust and immunity?", Volume 68, pp. 61–6.

Psychopaths are a necessary evil

D. Miric, A-M. Hallet-Mathieu and G. Amar, "Aetiology of antisocial personality disorder: Benefits for society from an evolutionary standpoint", Volume 65, pp. 665–70.

Cystic fibrosis is a legacy of the Black Death

W. F. Cassano, "Cystic fibrosis and the plague", Volume 18, pp. 51–2.

Modern toilets ruin legs

S. J. Sontag and J. N. Wanner, "The cause of leg cramps and knee pains: A hypothesis and effective treatment", Volume 25, pp. 35–41.

Queen Elizabeth I was part man

R. Bakan, "Queen Elizabeth I: A case of testicular feminization?", Volume 17, pp. 277–84.

Schizophrenia changed the course of English history

N. Bark, "Did schizophrenia change the course of English history? The mental illness of Henry VI", Volume 59, pp. 416–21.

Jesus, the Turin Shroud and spontaneous combustion

J. D. B. Clarkson, "A possible origin for the Turin shroud image", Volume 12, pp. 11–16.

Smoke made Neanderthals extinct

F. C. Størmer and I. Mysterud, "Cave smoke: Air pollution poisoning involved in Neanderthal extinction?", Volume 68, pp. 723–4.

English Sweating Disease was really anthrax

E. McSweegan, "Anthrax and the aetiology of the English Sweating Sickness", Volume 62, pp. 155–7.

Herrings saved us from heart disease

G. P. Walsh, "The history of the herring and with its decline the significance to health", Volume 20, pp. 133–7.

Gulf War Syndrome is an allergy to burgers

D. H. Hollander, "Beef allergy and the Persian Gulf syndrome", Volume 45, pp. 221–2.

Prehistoric fires protected man from lung cancer

S. M. Platek, G. G. Gallup and B. D. Fryer, "The fireside hypothesis: was there differential selection to tolerate air pollution during human evolution?", Volume 58, pp. 1–5.

Alfred Nobel was killed by dynamite

S. Sri Kantha, "Could nitroglycerine poisoning be the cause of Alfred Nobel's anginal pains and premature death?", Volume 49, pp. 303–6.

Why women groan during sex

T. Passie, U. Hartmann, U. Schneider and H. M. Emrich, "On the function of groaning and hyperventilation during sexual intercourse: intensification of sexual experience by altering brain metabolism through hippomania", Volume 60, pp. 660–63.

The importance of being impotent

O. N. Gofrit, "The evolutionary role of erectile dysfunction", Volume 67, pp. 1245–9.

Sex causes high blood pressure in pregnancy

G. F. Marx, S. H. Naushaba and H. Schulman, "Is pre-eclampsia a disease of the sexually active gravida?", Volume 7, pp. 1397–9.

Vasectomy lowers the risk of prostate cancer

A. R. Sheth and G. T. Panse, "Can vasectomy reduce the incidence of prostatic tumour?", Volume 8, pp. 237–41.

A cure for infatuation

M. M. Shoja, R. S. Tubbs and K. Ansarin, "A cure for infatuation? The potential 'therapeutic' role of pineal gland products such as melatonin and vasotocin in attenuating romantic love", Volume 68, pp. 1172–3.

Winter depression stops sex

J. M. Eagles, "Seasonal affective disorder: a vestigial evolutionary advantage?", Volume 63, pp. 767–72.

Gentlemen prefer blondes

V. S. Ramachandran, "Why do gentlemen prefer blondes?", Volume 48, pp. 19–20.

House smells turn teenage girls into women

J. Burger and M. Gochfeld, "A hypothesis on the role of pheromones on age of menarche", Volume 17, pp. 39–46.

Baby blues are caused by lack of sex

P. G. Ney, "The intravaginal absorption of male generated hormones and their possible effect on female behaviour", Volume 20, pp. 221–31.

Gum disease causes small babies

X. Xiong, P. Buekens, S. Vastardis and T. Wu, "Periodontal disease as one possible explanation for the Mexican paradox", Volume 67, pp. 1348–54.

Condoms increase the risk of breast cancer

A. N. Gjorgov, "Barrier contraceptive practice and male infertility as related factors to breast cancer in married women", Volume 4, pp. 79–88.

Sunny days make men violent

G. Schreiber, S. Avissar, Z. Tzahor, I. Barak-glantz and N. Grisaru, "Photoperiodicity and annual rhythms of wars and violent crimes", Volume 48, pp. 89–96.

The sun causes schizophrenia

R. C. Richardson-Andrews, "Sunspots and the recency theory of schizophrenia", Volume 44, pp. 16–19.

The sun fixes lifespan

G. E. Davis and W. E. Lowell, "Solar cycles and their relationship to human disease and adaptability", Volume 67, pp. 447–61.

Flu epidemics are affected by the sun

J. W. K. Yeung, "A hypothesis: Sunspot cycles may detect pandemic influenza A in 1700–2000 AD", Volume 67, pp. 1016–22.

Gout attacks are caused by the moon

M. Mikulecky and J. Rovensky, "Gout attacks and lunar cycle", Volume 55, pp. 24–5.

Chest pains are caused by the moon

M. Sok, M. Mikulecky and J. Erzen, "Onset of spontaneous pneumothorax and the synodic lunar cycle", Volume 57, pp. 638–41.

How weather affects mood

L. Sher, "Effects of the weather conditions on mood and behaviour: The role of acupuncture points", Volume 46, pp. 19–20.

Why Greenlanders have less cancer

T. C. Erren and C. Piekarski, "Does winter darkness in the Arctic protect against cancer? The melatonin hypothesis revisited", Volume 53, pp. 1–5.

Lights at night cause cancer

S. M. Pauley, "Lighting for the human circadian clock: recent research indicates that lighting has become a public health issue", Volume 63, pp. 588–96.

Dogs give women breast cancer

B. Laumbacher, B. Fellerhoff, B. Herzberger and R. Wank, "Do dogs harbour risk factors for human breast cancer?", Volume 67, pp. 21–6.

Electric typewriters cause breast cancer

S. Milham and E. Ossiander, "Electric typewriter exposure and increased female breast cancer mortality in typists", Volume 68, pp. 450–51.

Hairy people have less cancer

S. V. Komarova, "A moat around castle walls: The role of axillary and facial hair in lymph node protection from mutagenic factors", Volume 67, pp. 698–701.

Quitting smoking too fast triggers lung cancer

A. Kumar, K. Mallya and J. Kumar, "Are lung cancers triggered by stopping smoking?" Volume 68, pp. 1176–7.

Cancer is best diagnosed in the summer

A. Hykkerud Steindal, A. C. Porojnicu and J. Moan, "Is the seasonal variation in cancer prognosis caused by sun-induced folate degradation?", Volume 69, pp. 182–5.

Hairsprays cause cancer

M. Donovan, C. M. Tiwary, D. Axelrod, A. J. Sasco, L. Jones, R. Hajek, E. Sauber, J. Kuo and D. L. Davis, "Personal care products that contain estrogens or xenoestrogens may increase breast cancer risk," Volume 68, pp. 756–66.

Skin colour and breast cancer

J. T. Manning and N. Caswell, "Constitutive skin pigmentation: a marker of breast cancer risk?", Volume 63, pp. 787–9.

A cure for constipation

S. S. Hoseini and S. Gharibzadeh, "Squeezing the glans penis: A possible manoeuvre for improving the defecation process and preventing constipation", Volume 68, pp. 925–6.

Nuts cure toothache

C. Weber, "Eliminate infection (abscess) in teeth with cashew nuts", Volume 65, p. 1200.

Leather shoes cure diseases

A. A. Robinson, "Electrolysis between the feet and the ground and its probable health effects", Volume 5, pp. 1071–7.

A cure for hiccups

A. Kumar, "Gag reflex for arrest of hiccups", Volume 65, p. 1206.

Humming 120 times a day cures blocked noses

G. A. Eby, "Strong humming for one hour daily to terminate chronic rhinosinusitis in four days: A case report and hypothesis for action by stimulation of endogenous nasal nitric oxide production", Volume 66, pp. 851–4.

Magnets can make you taller

J. and A. Kumar. "Sustained repulsive magnetic force for bone lengthening", Volume 65, p. 630.

Drinking water lowers the risk of heart disease

R. K. Mathur, "The role of hypersomolal food in the development of atherosclerosis", Volume 64, pp. 579–81.

A cure for most diseases

H. Dehmelt, "Healthiest diet hypothesis: how to cure most diseases?", Volume 64, p. 882.

A cure for death

C. B. Olson, "A possible cure for death", Volume 26, pp. 77–84.

Pets prevent heart attacks

G. J. Patronek and L. T. Glickman, "Pet ownership protects against the risks and consequences of coronary heart disease", Volume 40, pp. 245–9.

Taking the elevator for a natural birth

B. Sabayan, A. Zolghadrasli and N. Mahmoudian, "Could taking an up-elevator on the way to the delivery room be a potential novel therapy for dystocia?", Volume 68, p. 227.

Seaweed may prevent AIDS

J. Teas, J. R. Hebert, J. Helen Fitton and P. V. Zimba, "Algae – a poor man's HAART?", Volume 62, pp. 507–10.

Worms prevent heart disease

E. Magen, G. Borkow, Z. Bentwich, J. Mishal and S. Scharf, "Can worms defend our hearts? Chronic helminthic infections may attenuate the development of cardiovascular diseases", Volume 64, pp. 904–9.

Killer viruses are hiding in the ice

A. W. Smith, D. E. Skilling, J. D. Castello and S. O. Rogers, "Ice as a reservoir for pathogenic human viruses: specifically, caliciviruses, influenza viruses, and enteroviruses", Volume 63, pp. 560–66.

Car travel causes heart disease

A. A. Robinson, "Heart disease, cancer and vehicle travel", Volume 5, pp. 323–8.

How soft drinks prevent stomach cancer

S. Seely, "The recession of gastric cancer and its possible causes", Volume 4, pp. 50–57.

Smoking caused rheumatoid arthritis

K. M. Fischer, "Hypothesis: Tobacco use is a risk factor in rheumatoid arthritis", Volume 34, pp. 116–17.

Tiny bugs living in the lungs cause asthma

H. van Woerden, "Dust mites living in human lungs – the cause of asthma?", Volume 63, pp. 193–7.

Killer popcorn

J. M. Blondell, "Pesticides and breast cancer, popcorn and colorectal cancer: Innovation versus fashion in dietary epidemiology", Volume 12, pp. 191–4.

Botox makes you thinner

E. C. H. Lim and R. C. S. Seet, "Botulinum toxin injections to reduce adiposity: Possibility, or fat chance?", Volume 67, pp. 1086–9.

Defecate at night to lose weight

N. Ahmad Aziz and M. Ibrahim Aziz, "Losing weight by defecating at night", Volume 67, p. 989.

Diet every other day to lose weight and live longer

J. B. Johnson, D. R. Laub and S. John, "The effect on health of alternate day calorie restriction: Eating less and more than needed on alternate days prolongs life", Volume 67, pp. 209–11.

Salt, the cocaine of the kitchen?

Y. Tekol, "Salt addiction: A different kind of drug addiction", Volume 67, pp. 1233–4.

Why American heads are getting smaller (and the French bigger)

N. Moishezon-Blank, "Commentary on the possible effect of hormones in food on human growth", Volume 38, pp. 273–7.

Eating pork causes multiple sclerosis

A. A. Nanji, and S. Narod, "Multiple sclerosis, latitude and dietary fat: Is pork the missing link?", Volume 20, pp. 279–82.

Mad flour disease

C. A. Shaw and J. S. Bains, "Did consumption of flour bleached by the agene process contribute to the incidence of neurological disease?", Volume 51, pp. 477–81.

Milk causes cancer

D. Ganmaa, X. M. Li, L. Q. Qin, P. Y. Wang, M. Takeda and A. Sato, "The experience of Japan as a clue to the aetiology of testicular and prostatic cancers", Volume 60, pp. 724–30.

Rats spread mad cow disease to humans

G. P. Concepcion and E. A. Padlan, "Are humans getting 'mad-cow disease' from eating beef, or something else?", Volume 60, pp. 699–701.

How a prescription drug increased depression in children

A. Agus, S. Surja and R. S. El-Mallakh, "Fertility and childhood bipolar disorder", in press.

MS and the domestic cat

R. D. Cook, "Multiple sclerosis: Is the domestic cat involved?", Volume 7, pp. 147–54.

Soap causes heart disease

R. H. Cane, "The role of soap and nutrition in producing human diseases", Volume 11, pp. 251–4.

Autism and city life

F. H. Previc, "Prenatal influences on brain dopamine and their relevance to the rising incidence of autism", Volume 68, pp. 46–60.

Power lines cause depression

D. L. Henshaw, "Does our electricity distribution system pose a serious risk to public health?", Volume 59, pp. 39–51.

Heeled shoes cause schizophrenia

J. Flensmark, "Is there an association between the use of heeled footwear and schizophrenia?", Volume 63, pp. 740–47.

Fluoride makes teeth crooked

P. R. N. Sutton, "Can water fluoridation increase orthodontic problems?", Volume 26, pp. 63–4.

Rain causes blood clots

R. Clauss, J. Mayes, P. Hilton and R. Lawrenson, "The influence of weather and environment on pulmonary embolism: pollutants and fossil fuels", Volume 64, pp. 1198–1201.

Climate change caused diabetes

S. Moalem, K. B. Storey, M. E. Percy, M. C. Peros and D. P. Perl, "The sweet thing about Type 1 diabetes: A cryoprotective evolutionary adaptation", Volume 65, pp. 8–16.

TV shows cause dementia

M. Aronson, "Does excessive television viewing contribute to the development of dementia?", Volume 41, pp. 465–6.

Stress can seriously damage your teeth

P. R. N. Sutton, "Psychosomatic dental disease: Is mental stress in adults followed by acute dental caries in all racial groups?", Volume 41, pp. 279–81.

Gloves cause asthma

J. Worth, "Neonatal sensitization to latex", Volume 54, pp. 29–33.

ABOUT THE AUTHOR

ROGER DOBSON is an award-winning freelance journalist who contributes to a number of national newspapers on health and science, including the *Daily Mail*, *The Times* and the *Sunday Times*, and the *Independent* and *Independent on Sunday*, as well as the *British Medical Journal*. He and his family live on the slopes of the Skirrid mountain near Abergavenny in Monmouthshire, South Wales.